Wolf Matriarchs of Yellowstone

The beginning of a new wolf era

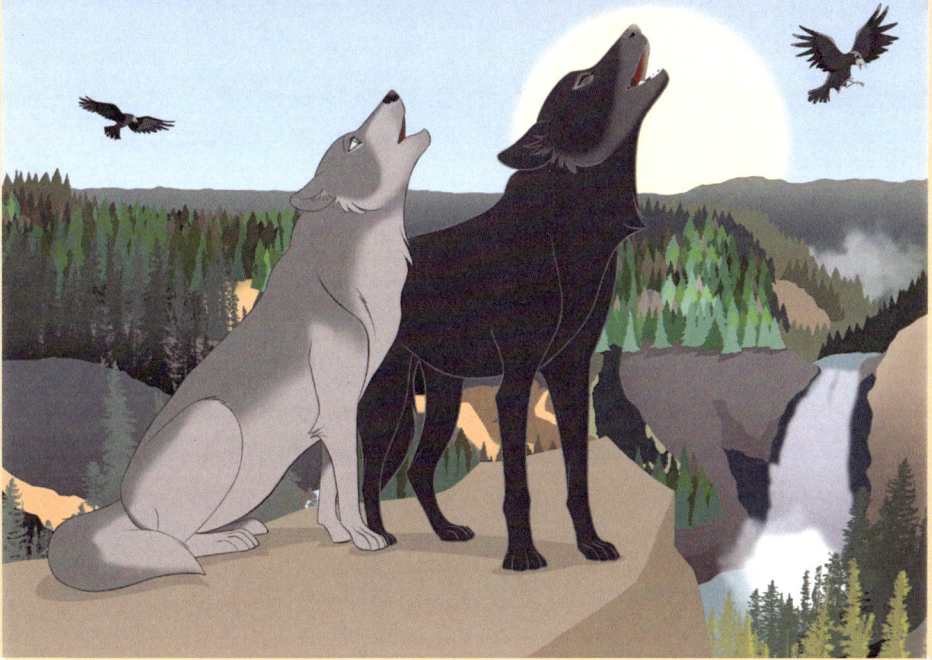

By Sylvia M. Medina and
Douglas W. Smith

Illustrations by Andreas Wessel-Therhorn

green kids club

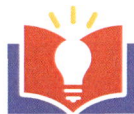

Noah Text®

Noah Text®

The **Noah Text®** Chapter Books have been carefully selected and curated to meet the needs of all readers – and striving and struggling readers in particular – by providing superior text accessibility. Noah Text® books are rendered in **Noah Text®, a patented evidence-based methodology for displaying text that increases reading skill.**

Grounded in the science of reading, Noah Text® is a specialized scaffolded text that shows **syllable patterns** within words by highlighting them with bold and unbold and marking **long vowels** (vowels that "say their own names"). Here are some examples:

entertainment	⇨	**en**ter**tain**ment
beautiful	⇨	**bea**uti**ful**
photosynthesis	⇨	**ph**oto**syn**the**sis**
comprehension	⇨	**com**pre**hen**sion
ironic	⇨	**i**ron**ic**
lieutenant	⇨	**lie**uten**ant**
achievement	⇨	**a**chieve**ment**
epitome	⇨	**e**pito**me**
ideology	⇨	**i**de**ol**ogy
coordination	⇨	**co**ordi**na**tion

By showing readers the structure of words, Noah Text® enhances reading skills, freeing up cognitive resources that readers can devote to comprehension. Noah Text® simulates simpler writing systems (e.g., Finland's) in which learning to read is easier due to visible, predictable word patterns. As a result, Noah Text® increases reading fluency, stamina, accuracy, and confidence while building skills that transfer to plain text reading.

Highly recommended by structured literacy specialists, Noah Text® is effective for developing, struggling, and dyslexic readers and for multilingual learners. Noah Text® enables resistant and struggling readers to advance their reading skills beyond basic proficiency so that they can tackle higher-level learning.

Readers find Noah Text® intuitive and easy to use, requiring little to no instruction to get started. A sound key that further explains how Noah Text® works can be found at the back of this book.

For further information on Noah Text® and its products, please visit www.noahtext.com.

Dear Parents, Educators, and Striving English-Language Readers,

As individuals develop the ability to read beyond the elementary level, their challenge is to build on a basic awareness of how patterns of letters stand for sounds and how those sounds come together to make words. Readers who learn the letter patterns in one-syllable words are poised to recognize them in longer, multisyllable words.

For struggling readers, however, long words can appear to be a sea of individual letters whose syllable sub-divisions are hard to discern. This series from Noah Text® highlights where syllable breaks occur, while also signaling long vowels -- those that "say their own names."   These visual cues help struggling readers decode words more easily and read more fluently and accurately.

Now, with Noah Text® Chapter Books, all individuals can learn to read with less effort, empowering them to experience enriching literature and enlightening informational texts.

Miriam Cherkes-Julkowski, Ph.D.
Professor, Educational Psychology (retired)
Educational Diagnostician and Consultant

About the Author - Sylvia M. Medina is the president, primary author, and creative lead of the Green Kids Club. She has spent her career focused on environmental issues and helping to preserve animal welfare. She hopes to teach children the importance of helping to save our world and its animals.

Yellowstone's Senior Wildlife Biologist and Wolf Project leader - Douglas W. Smith His original job was as the Project Leader for the Yellowstone Wolf Project which involved the reintroduction and restoration of wolves to Yellowstone National Park. He has produced five books, "Decade of the Wolf," "Yellowstone Wolves," "Wolves on the Hunt," "Yellowstone Birds," and "The Wolves of Yellowstone."

About the Illustrator - Andreas Wessel-Therhorn is from Münster, Germany. He has been working in animation for more than 32 years for, among others, Walt Disney Feature Animation, Warner Bros., and credits include Hercules, Tarzan, Fantasia 2000, and Mary Poppins Returns.

Our collaborator - Yellowstone Forever's mission is to protect, preserve, and enhance Yellowstone National Park through educational and philanthropy. www.yellowstone.org

We want to acknowledge the input from ~ Yellowstone Park Service - Photo Collection. Special thanks to Tin Man Lee, Trent Sizemore, and Julie Argyle for wonderful photos.

Contributors - Leo Leckie, Jon Potter, Jim Halfpenny, Charlotte Broussard, Jadon Schemers, Bruce Miller, Tiago Miller, and Joy Eagle

green kids club
www.greenkidsclub.com

Wolf Matriarchs of Yellowstone

The beginning of a new wolf era

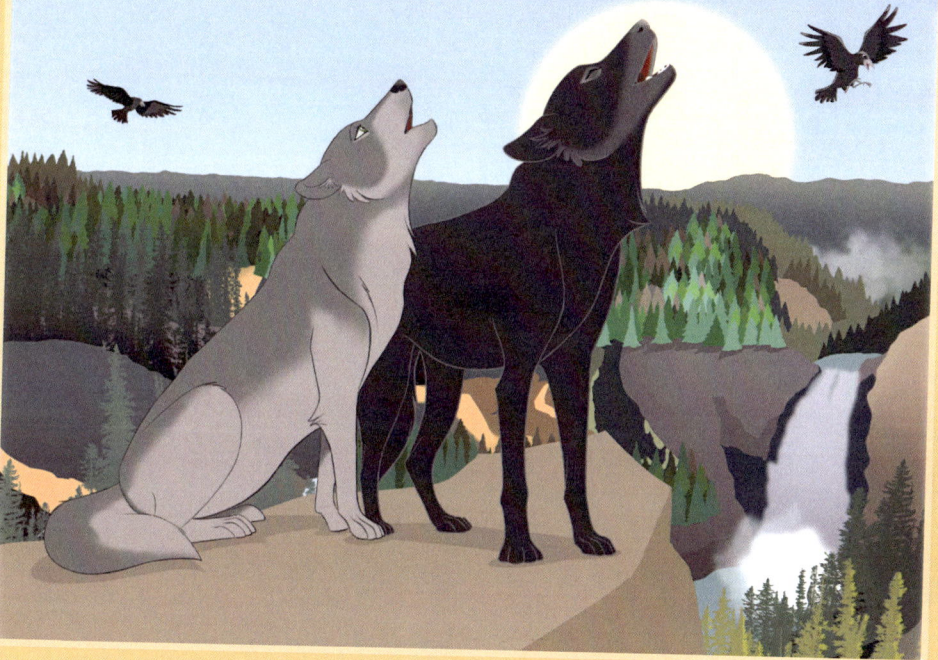

By Sylvia M. Medina and
Douglas W. Smith

Illustrations by Andreas Wessel-Therhorn

green kids club

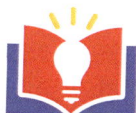

Noah Text®

CONTENTS

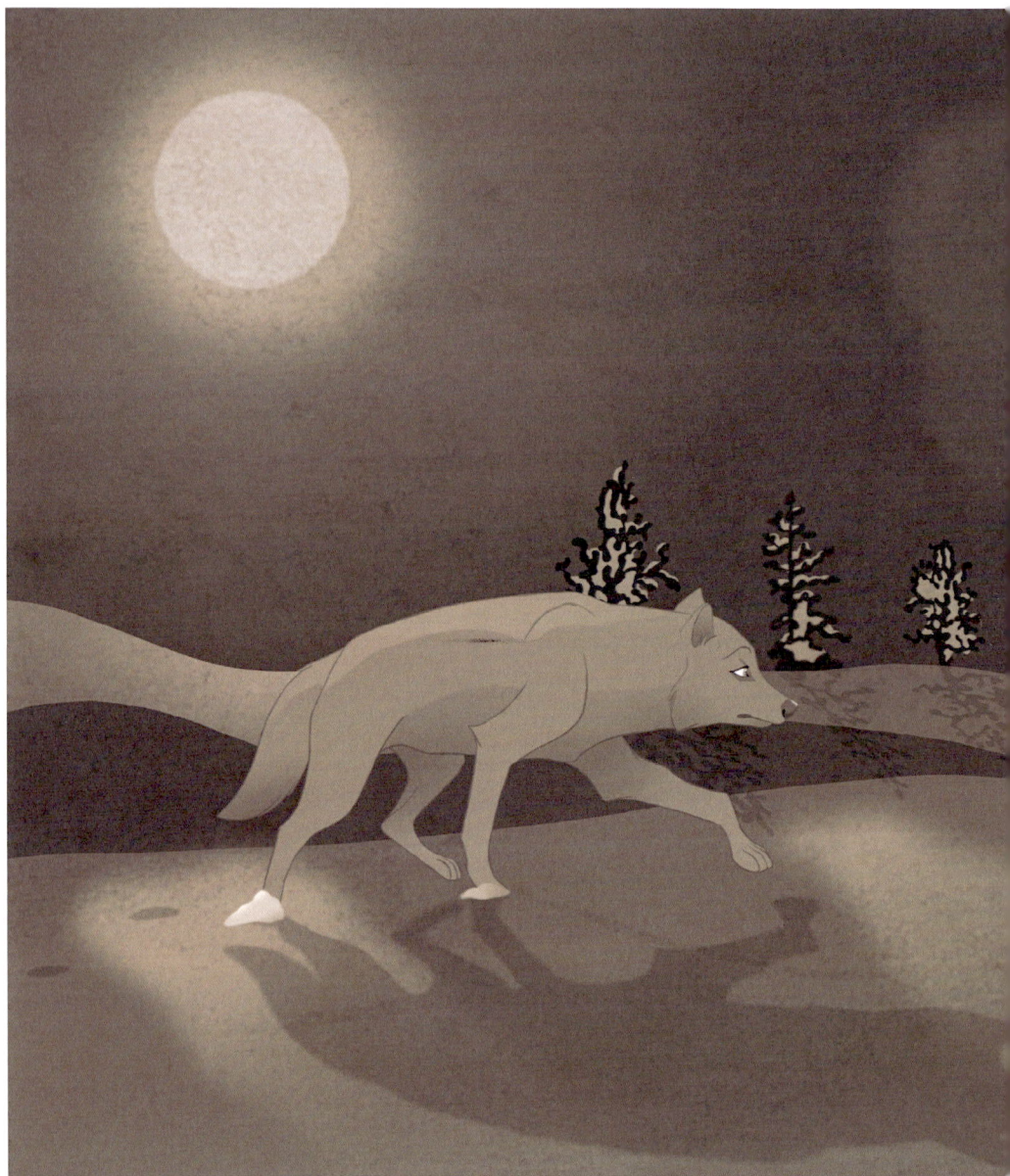

Early **Yell**o**wst**o**ne** and Wolves

The moon sh_o_ne **br**i**ght**ly on the **glis**ten**ing** wh_i_te sn_o_w as the wolf **qu**i**etly pad**ded thro_u_gh the **crust**ed _i_ce field. H_e_ was **trav**el**ing** to the spot where h_e_ last saw his m_a_te. H_e_ **could**n't f_i_nd her – or **an**y**one**. H_e_ had been **walk**ing for d_a_ys, **mov**ing from **val**l_e_y to **val**l_e_y in **Yell**o**wst**o**ne**.

1

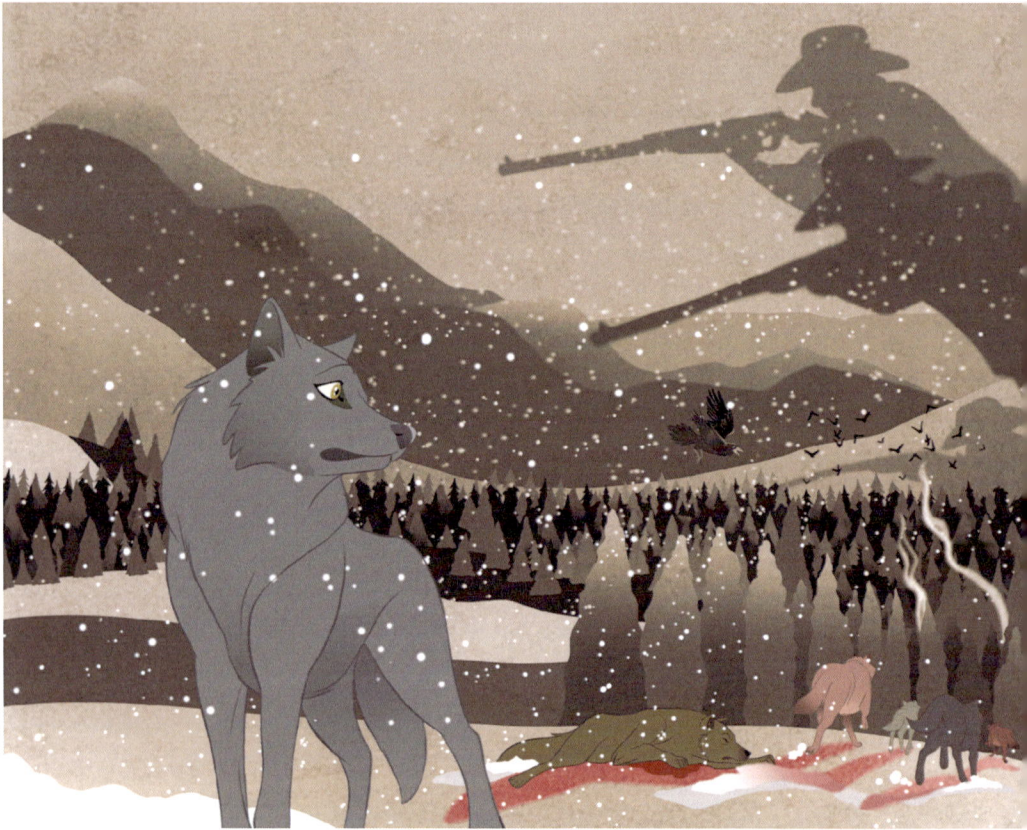

The last time he heard from his pack was right **be**fore he heard the **a**larm**ing** sounds of crack, crack, crack **com**ing from the **di**rec**tion** of his **fam**ily.

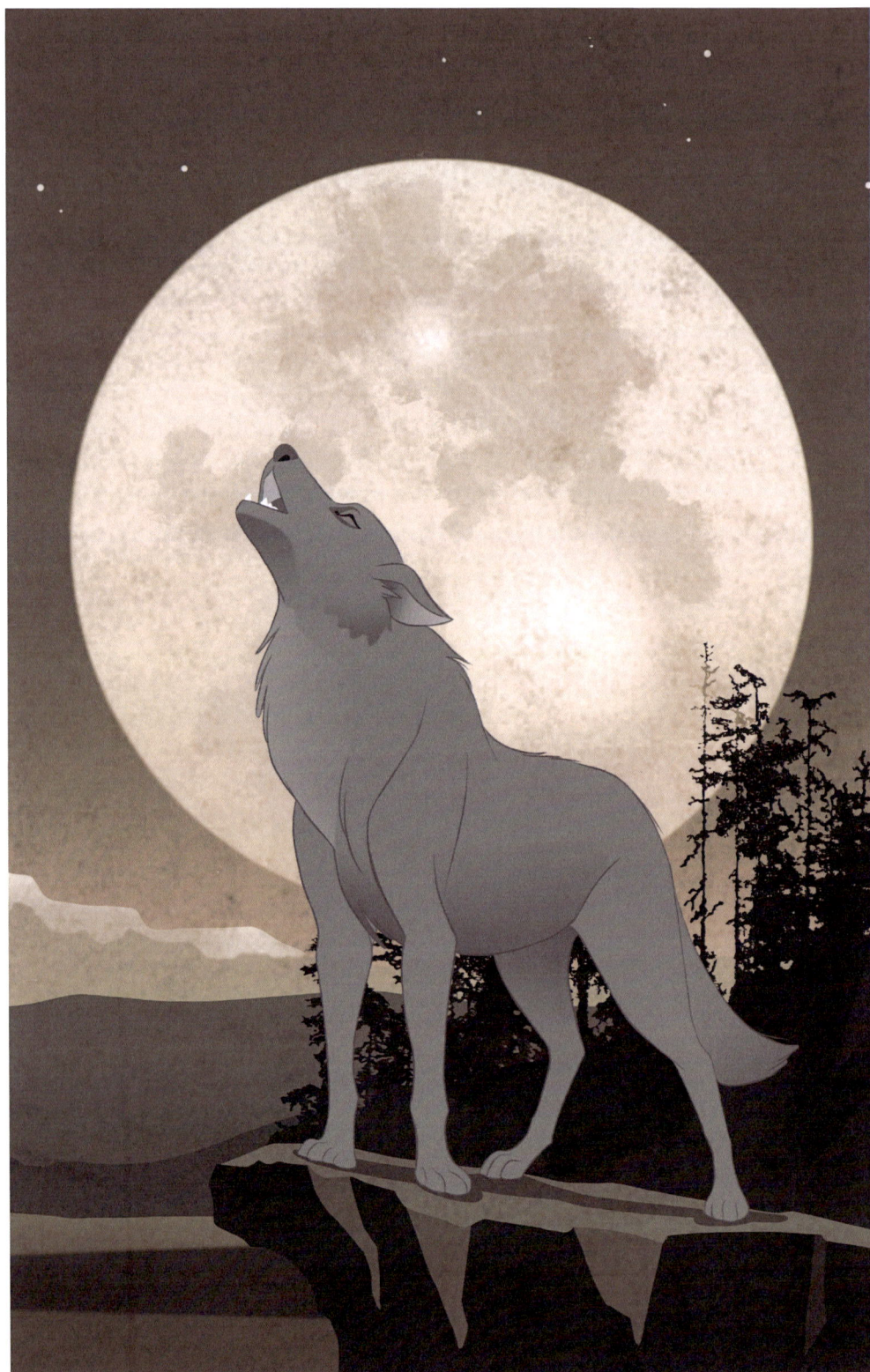

He sat **qui**etly on the ledge, over the **beau**ti**ful La**mar **Val**ley – his home. He was all **a**lone. He **be**gan **howl**ing – first **soft**ly, then **loud**er, and then even **loud**er still. **Af**ter a **mo**ment, he stopped **hop**ing to hear a **re**ply but only **si**lence **gree**ted him. The wolf looked back **sor**rowful**ly** at the last spot where he had last seen his **fam**ily. He let out one more howl and ran out of **Yel**low**stone**, in search of his **part**ner.

He was **ut**ter**ly a**lone.

The last of his kind.

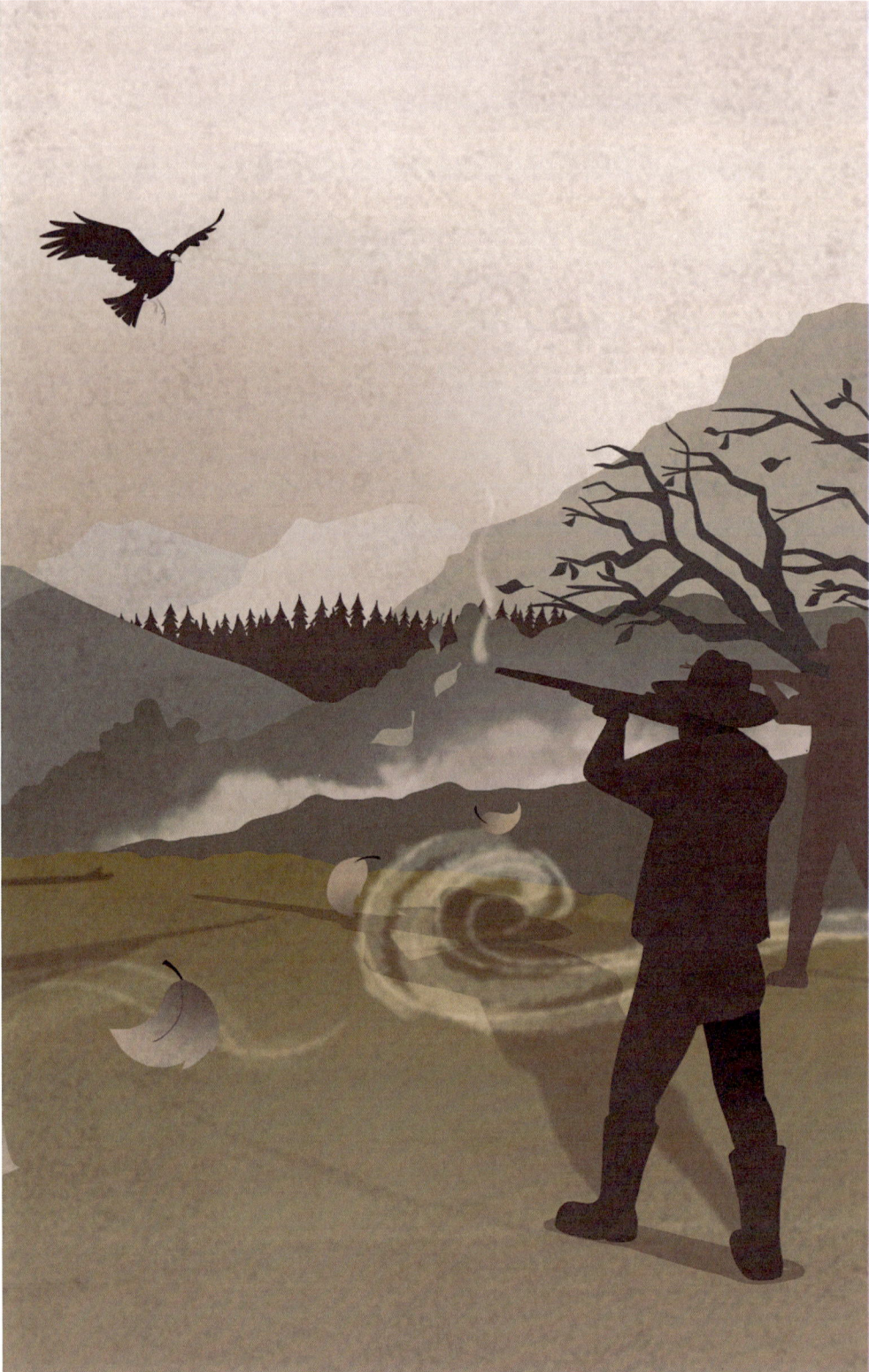

By 1926, the last of the wolves had either left or been **ex**ter**mi**n<u>a</u>**ted**, and none were s<u>ee</u>n for **de**c<u>a</u>des. The wolves were killed **be**cause **hu**mans did not l<u>i</u>ke the wolves. They felt they were **ta**king too **man**y of the d<u>ee</u>r and elk **pop**ul<u>a</u>tions. **Man**y al**s<u>o</u>** thought the wolves were **prey**ing on their **l<u>i</u>ve**stock, and that by **e**rad**ic**<u>at</u>**ing** the wolves, they could **pr<u>o</u>**tect their **an**i**mals**. This shift in the **ec<u>o</u>sys**tem **cr<u>ea</u>ted** an **im**bal**ance**, **l<u>ea</u>d**ing to an **in**cr<u>ea</u>se in the d<u>ee</u>r and **oth**er **un**g<u>u</u>late **pop**ul<u>a</u>tions d<u>ue</u> to the lack of wolves.

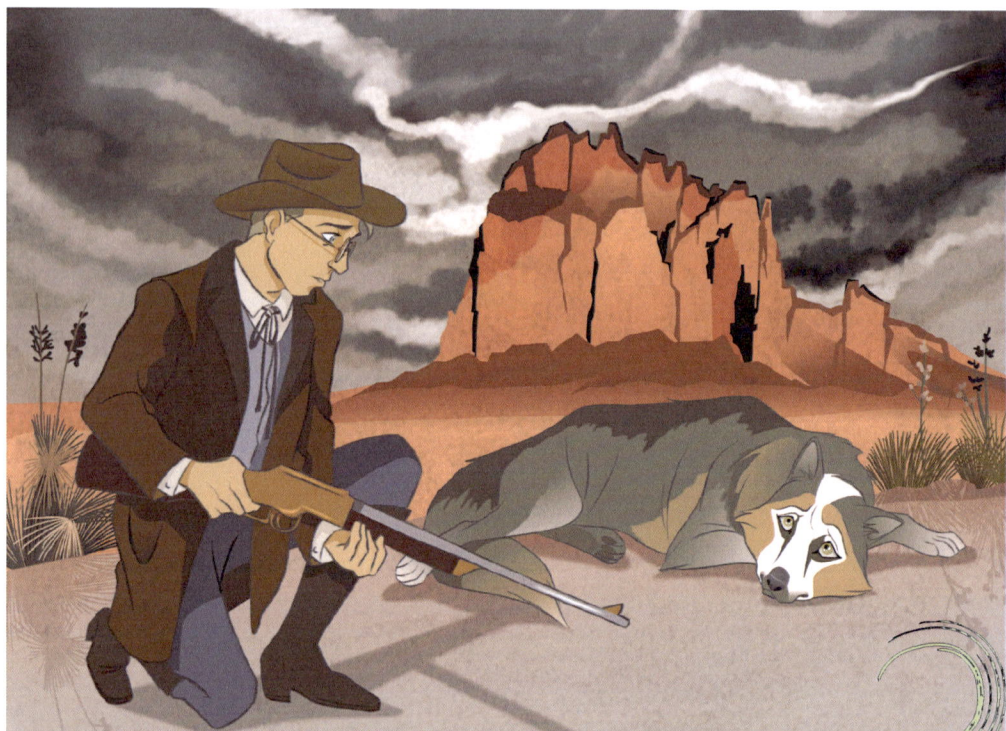
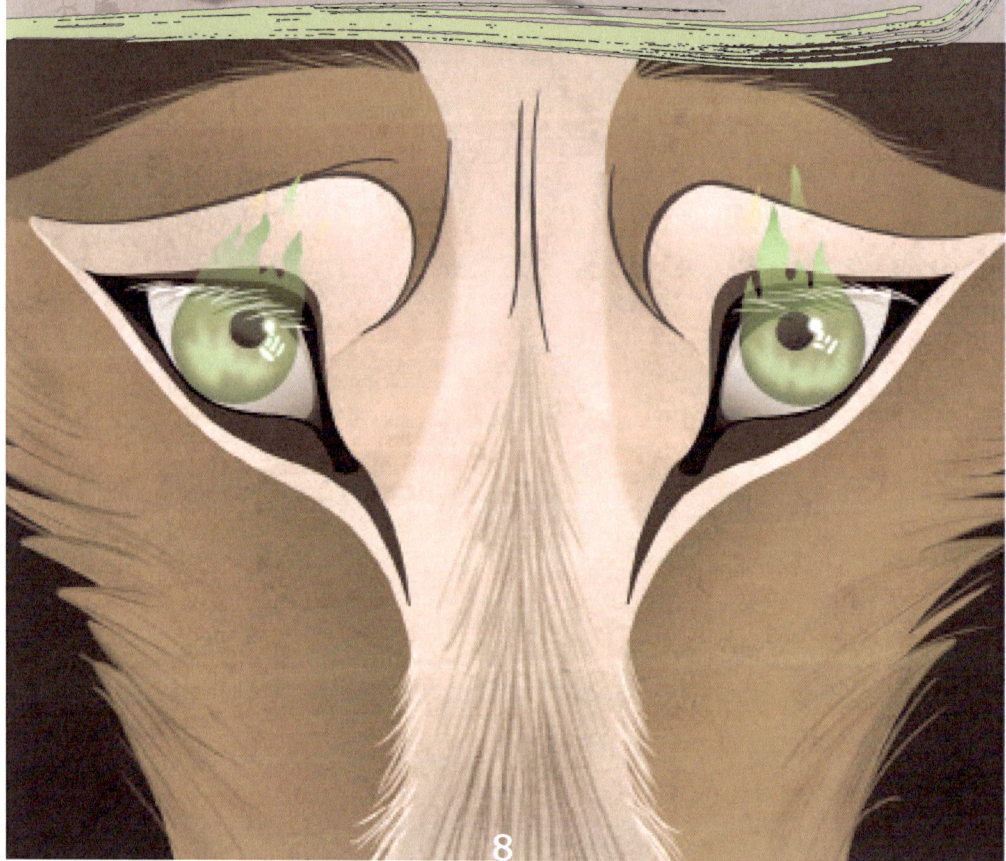

Chapter 2

Ald**o** **Le**op**o**ld and the **En**dan**g**ered S**pe**ci**e**s Act

In 1930, a man n**a**med **Al**d**o** **Le**op**o**ld was **hunt**ing in New **Mex**ic**o**. H**e** **dis**liked wolves, **think**ing they were a **men**ace, and **want**ed to rid the **ar**e**a** of all of them. Wh**i**le **hunt**ing for d**ee**r, h**e** **spot**ted a **fe**m**a**le wolf.

Imm**e**di**a**tel**y**, h**e** shot her.

Exc**i**ted, h**e** ran **o**ver to her as sh**e** l**a**y **dy**ing. When h**e** r**e**ached her, sh**e** **lift**ed her head and looked str**ai**ght **in**to his eyes. Her gr**ee**n eyes **glim**mered as sh**e** g**a**zed d**ee**p **in**to him, and at that **mo**ment h**e** knew.

*H**e** watched the **o**ld wolf as the fi**e**rce gr**ee**n fi**r**e d**i**ed in her eyes.*

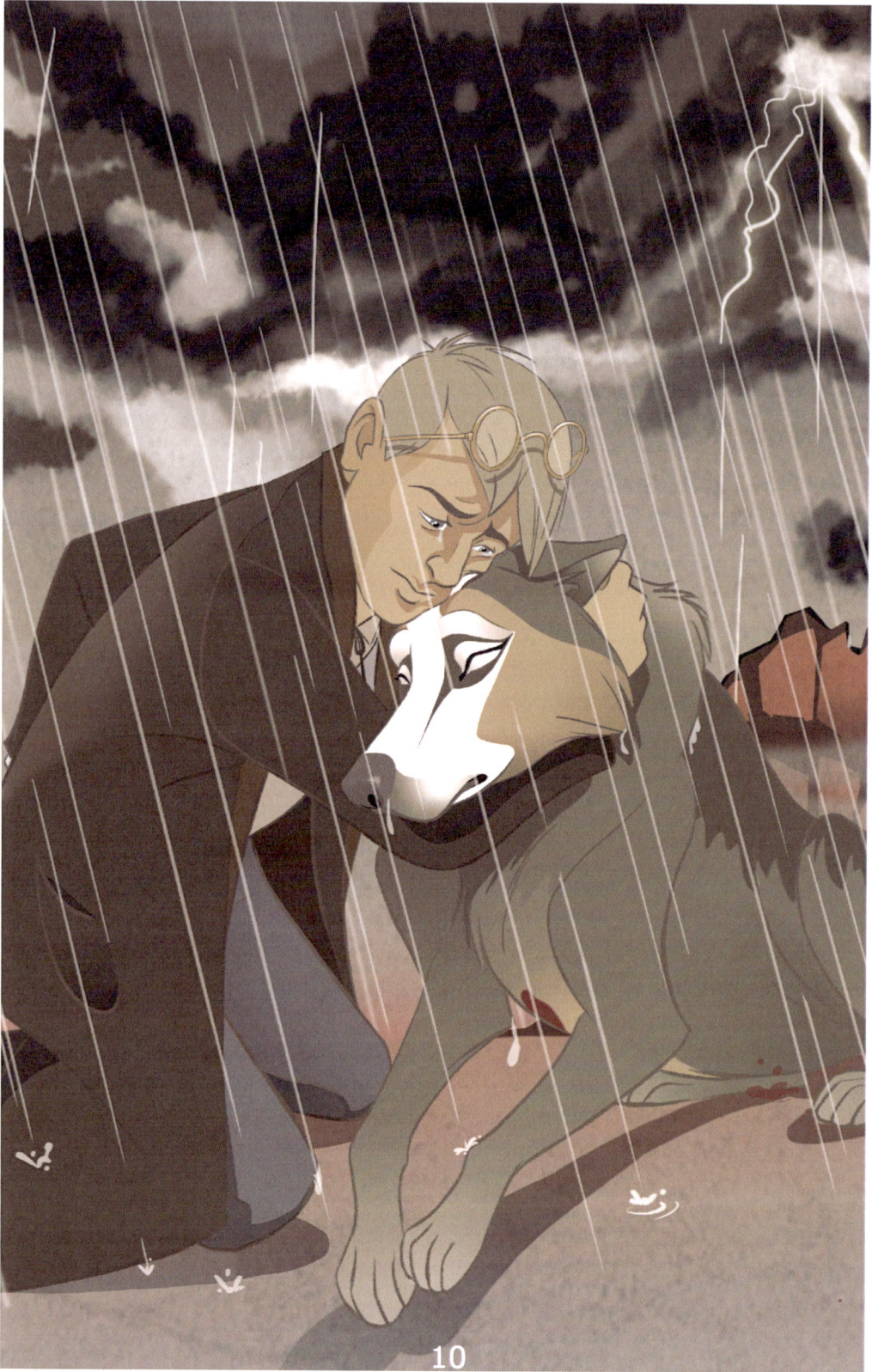

She then closed her eyes and was no more. **Le**o**pol**d fell to his knees, **weep**ing as he looked at the wolf he had killed. The look she gave him made him **re**al**ize** that he had to stop the **de**struc**tion** of the wolves caused by **hu**mans' **ac**tions **driv**en by **so**ci**etal forc**es.

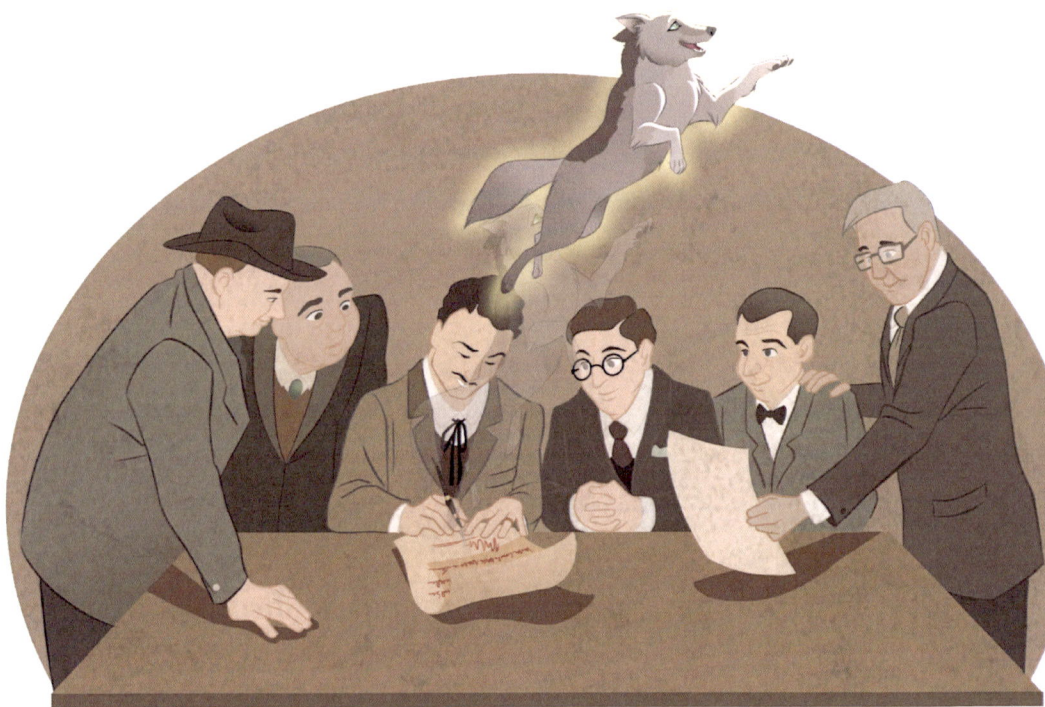

In 1994, **in**spired by the words of **con**serva**tion**ist **Al**do **Le**opold, groups of people conven**ed** to **dis**cuss the reintro**duction** of wolves **in**to **Yel**lowstone. The **bi**ologists and **oth**er **ex**perts **in**volved knew it was time to bring the wolf back. The **En**dan**gered Sp**ecies Act (**ESA**) was **en**act**ed**, pav**ing** the way for **re**intro**ducing** wolves and **oth**er sp**ec**ies back **in**to their **na**tive lands. The **ESA** aims to stop the **ex**tinc**tion** of plants and **an**imals caused by **hu**man **ac**tions. The list works like an 'emer**gen**cy room' for **threat**ened plants and **an**imals with the hope that those placed on the list will **e**ven**tu**ally re**cov**er and no **long**er be **con**sid**ered** en**dan**gered.

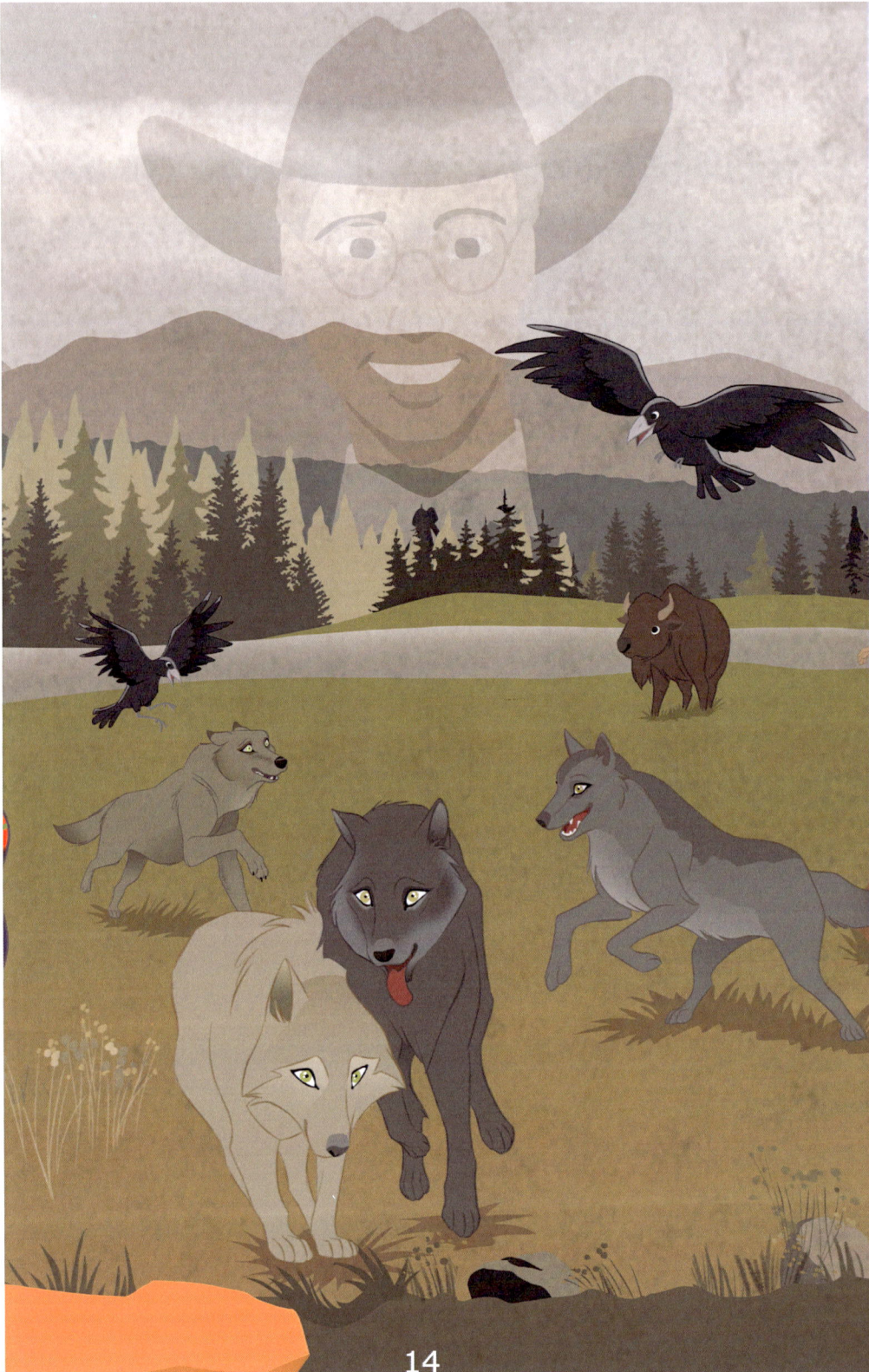

Many **na**tive **peo**ple and **oth**er wolf **sup**port**ers** were thrilled that the wolves were **re**turn**ing**. **Le**op**o**ld**'s** **vi**sion was **com**ing tr**u**e.

Oper**a**tion **Wolf**stock had **be**gun!

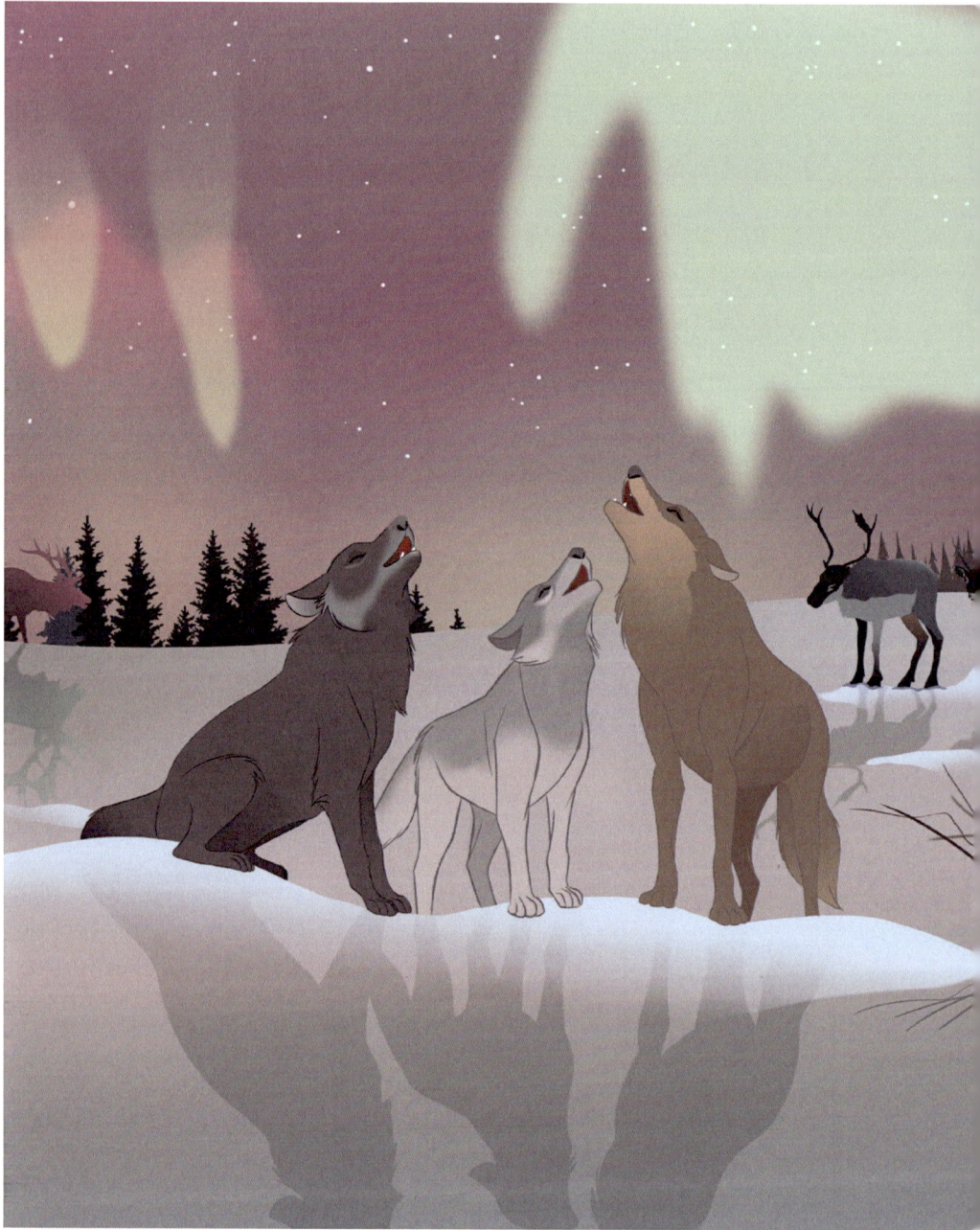

Bringing the Wolves Back!

While in **Canada**, a **fam**ily of three wolves played in the snow, **un**der the bright lights of the **aur**ora **bor**ealis. This was a small pack or **fam**ily of wolves with a **moth**er, **fa**ther and their **daugh**ter. There were **plen**ty of elk and deer for the wolves to hunt and feed on. The land was wild, and the **win**ters were cold and harsh – **per**fect for wolves as they love the cold, which is where they evolved.

The wolves stopped **play**ing and **start**ed **howl**ing to let **oth**er wolves know that this was their **terri**tory. A few **mi**nutes **la**ter, they heard the **dis**tant howls of **an**oth**er** pack of wolves **howl**ing back, through the **fro**zen cold **land**scape.

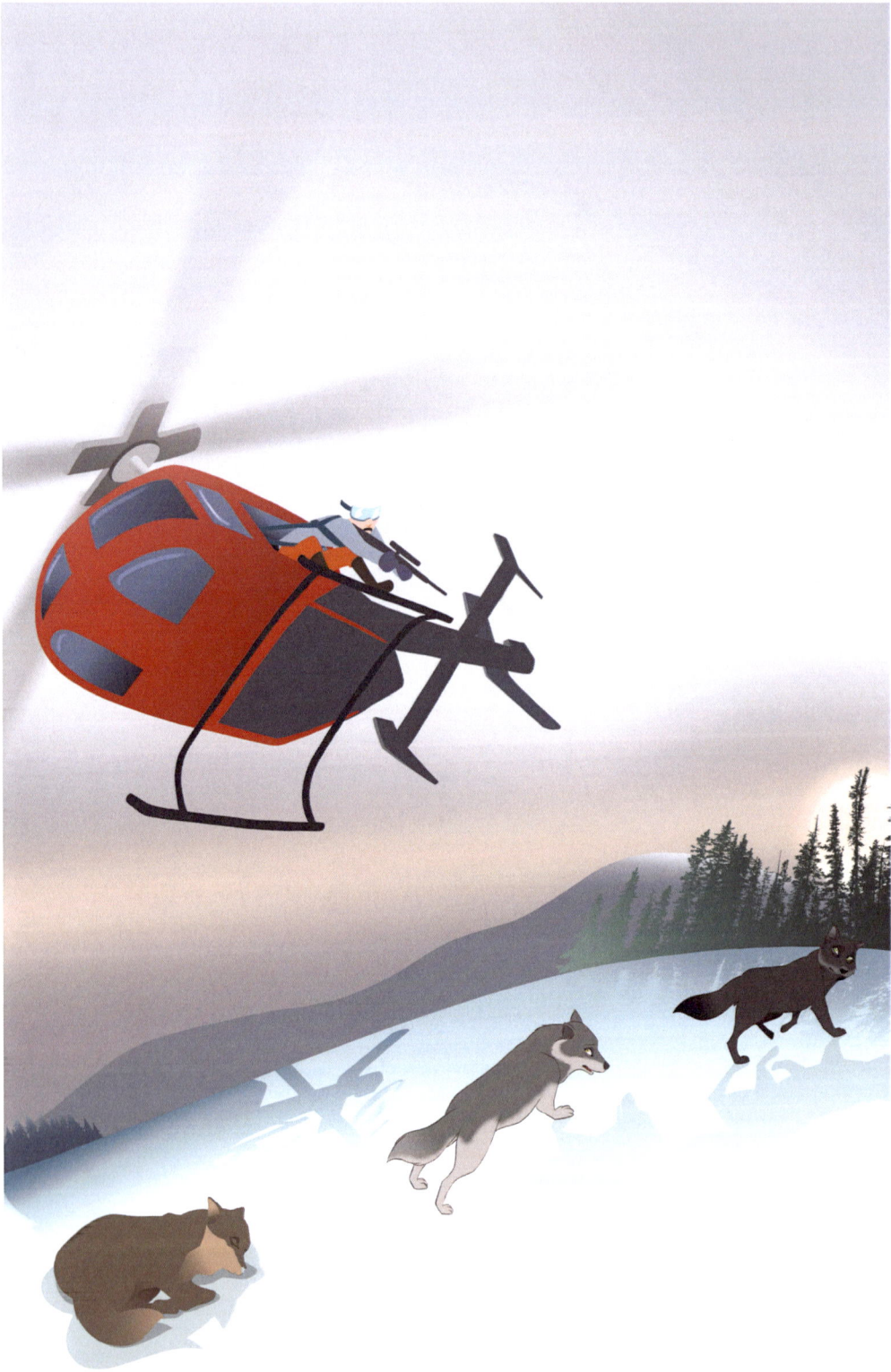

The **fam**ily curled up to sleep – with the **moth**er and **fa**ther wolf and their young **daug**hter **be**side them. As they slept, they **occa**sionally heard **howl**ing from **a**far; the **moth**er wolf would stand up and howl back.

Sud**denly,** the wolves heard a loud noise **com**ing from the sky. The wolves jumped up and **start**ed to run. The **moth**er wolf led the way, with her **daugh**ter foll**owing** cl**ose**ly **be**hind her. **Run**ning through the snow, she looked up **to**wards the noise and saw a man with a big **mus**tache **lean**ing down, **hold**ing **some**thing in his hands.

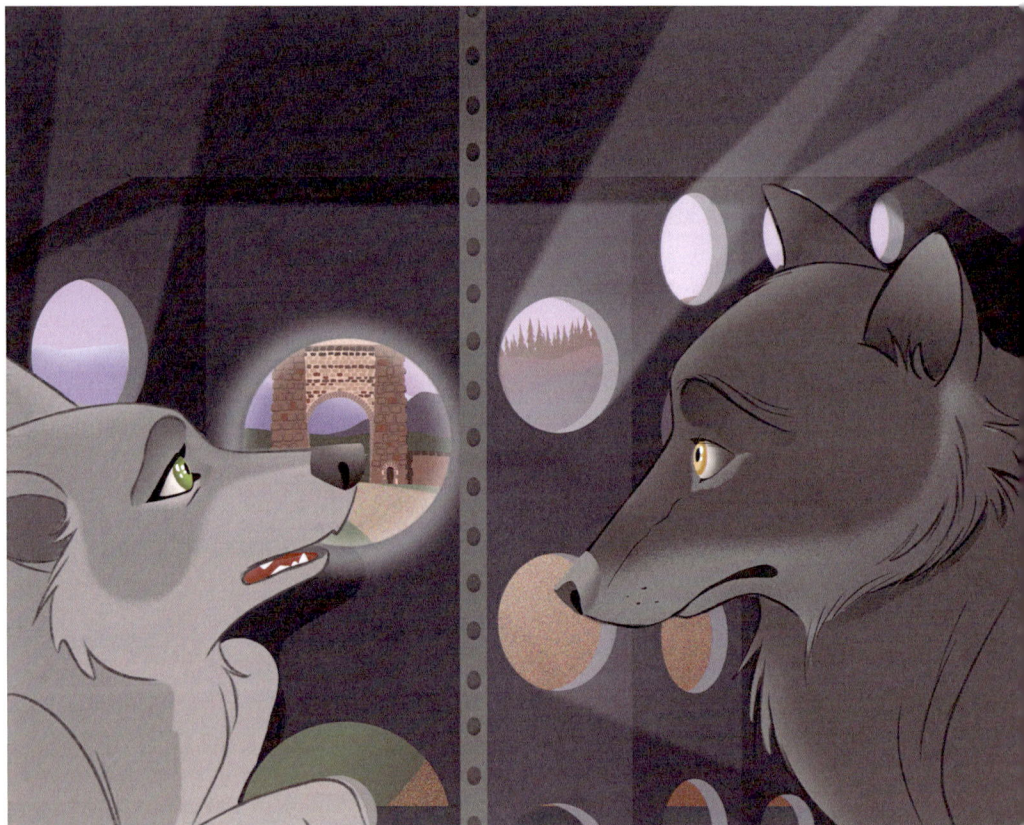

That was the last sh**e** **re**mem**bered** **be**fore **wa**king up to f**i**nd **her**self in a box-l**i**ke cr**a**te.

Next to her, sh**e** heard **whi**ning from **an**oth**er** cr**a**te and knew it was her **daugh**ter. Sh**e**, too, had been caught. The **moth**er wolf **whim**pered, and sh**e** heard her **daugh**ter **whim**per back, but sh**e** did not h**ea**r her m**a**te **re**spond. H**e** was not with them. Their **fami**ly had been torn **a**part, and sh**e** **nev**er saw him **a**gain.

The wolves were **trans**port**ed** by **a**ir to their new h**o**me. They looked out the cr**a**te **win**d**o**ws, and **see**ing **e**ach **oth**er was **com**fort**ing**, but they were still sc**a**red.

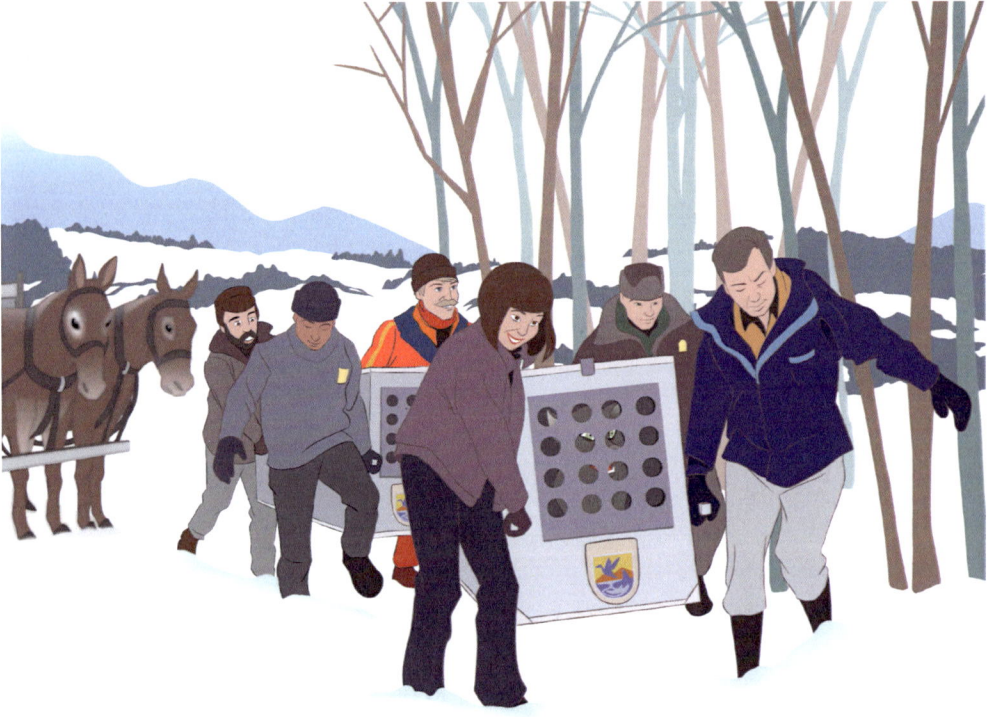

The wolves **re**mained in their crates **un**til two men **lift**ed the **box**es and placed them on a **trail**er pulled by mules.

The **moth**er wolf smelled the cold, **snow**y air - which had an **un**familiar scent, but the **sur**round**ings** looked like her old home.

When the mules came to a stop, **In**terior **Sec**retary Bruce **Bab**bitt and **Mol**lie **Beat**tie, the first **fe**male **Direc**tor of the U.S. Fish **& Wild**life **Ser**vice, **lift**ed and **car**ried the crates **in**to the **en**clo**sure**.

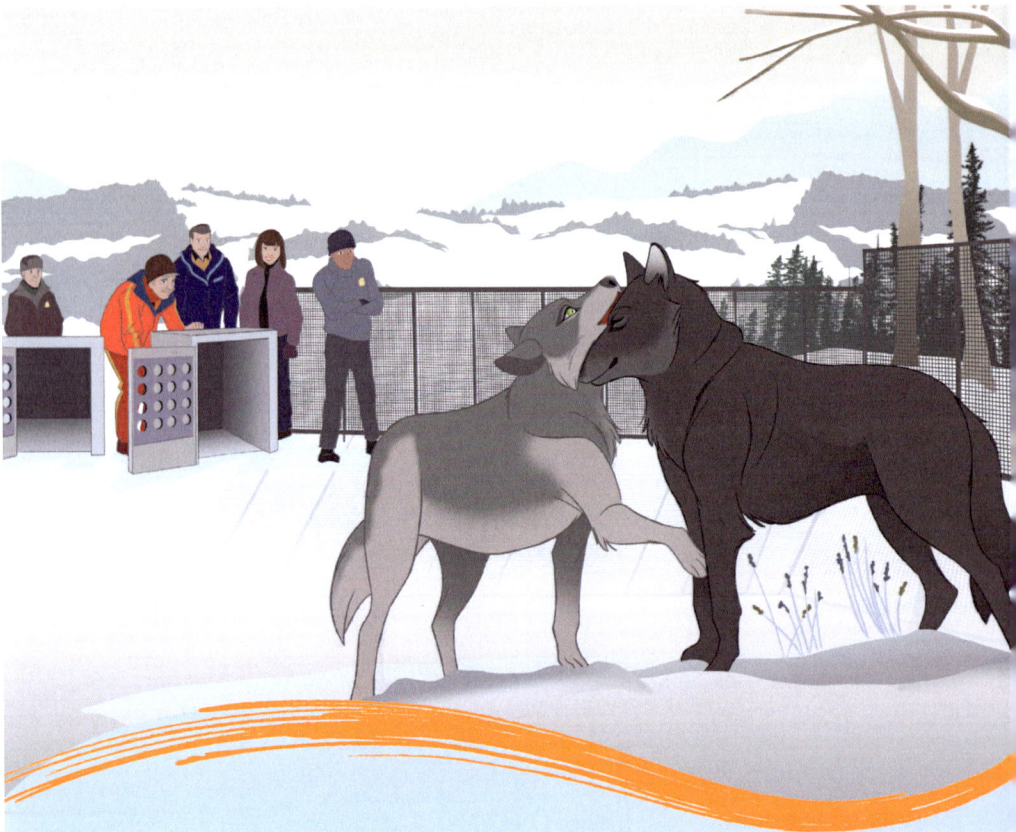

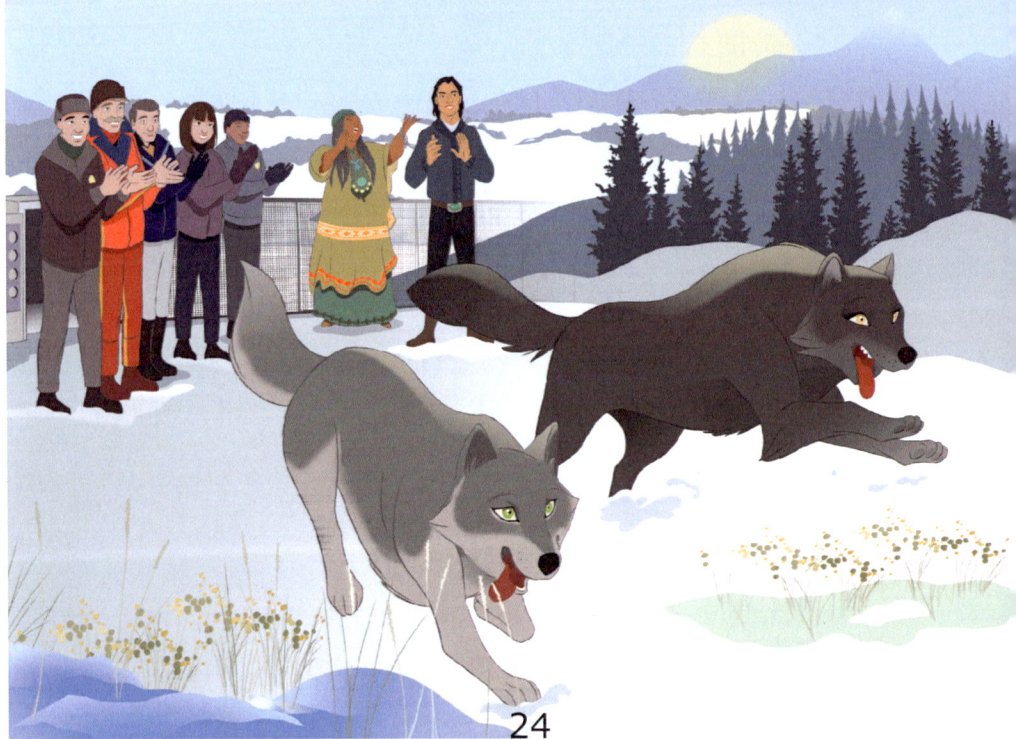

The man with the big **mus**tache **ap**pr**o**ached her cr**a**te and **o**pened the door. The **moth**er wolf saw the **o**pen door and ran out as fast as **pos**si**ble** but was stopped by a fence. **Un**a**ble** to g**o** **an**y **fur**ther, sh**e** looked up and saw her **daugh**ter **run**ning **to**wards her. The two wolves rushed to m**ee**t **e**ach **oth**er, **joy**fully **lick**ing and **nuz**zling one **an**oth**er**. The **moth**er had black fur, while her daughter had gr**a**y.

Then they heard a str**a**nge sound **com**ing from the crowd. The **pe**o**o**ple were **clap**ping their hands and **smi**l**i**ng **proud**ly.

THE WOLVES WERE BACK!

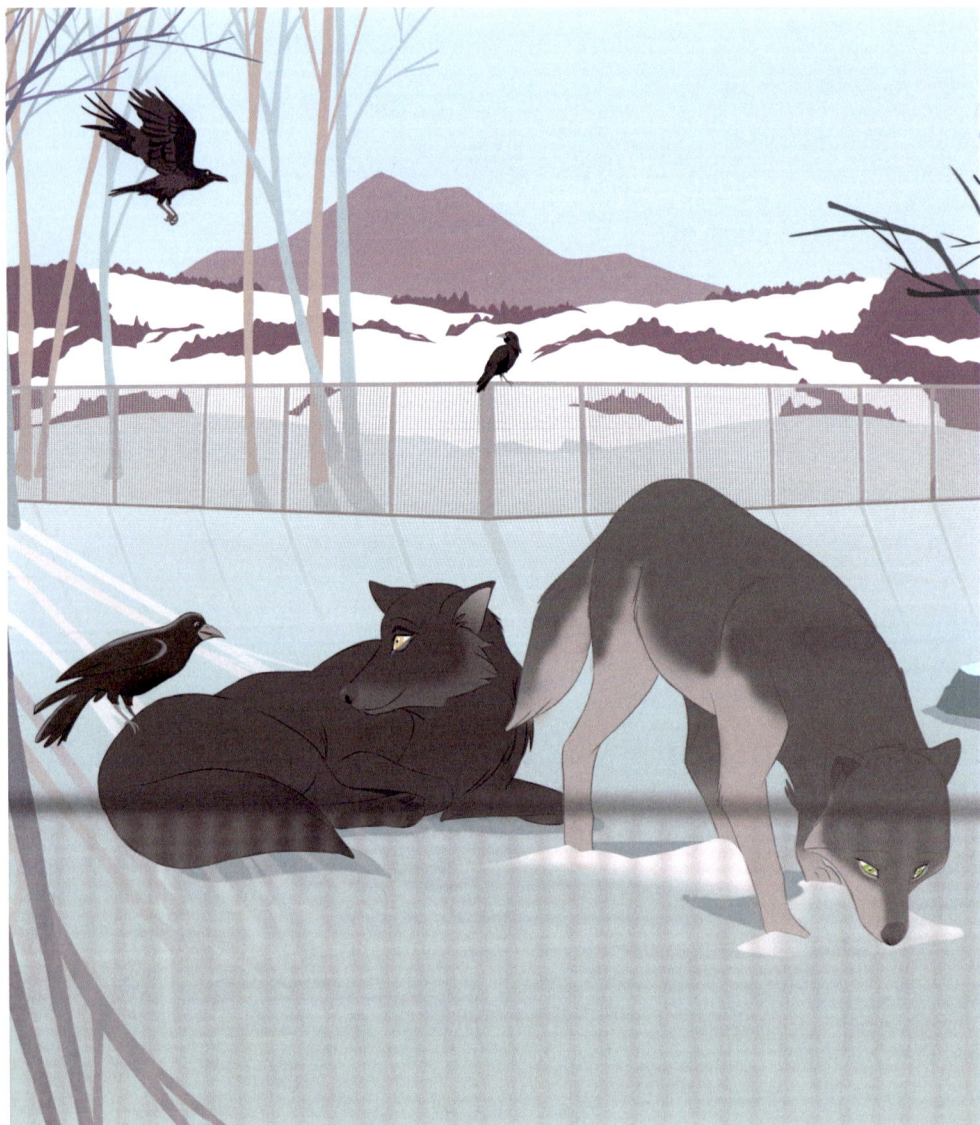

The Rose Creek Wolf **Family**

Most **peo**ple left while the **moth**er wolf and her **daugh**ter **ad**justed to their new **sur**round**ings**. Their new home was a round fence or **en**clo**sure** with a pen in the back called an **ac**climation pen. The wolves were not **giv**en names; **in**stead, the **Na**tion**al** Park **as**signed them **num**bers, which is how they would be known. This was done to try to **pre**vent **peo**ple from **fee**ling a sense of **own**ership or **an**thro**po**mor**phiz**ing the **an**imals. The **moth**er wolf was **giv**en the **num**ber 9, while the **daugh**ter **re**ceived the **num**ber 7. **Some**times, the **work**ers would come and bring them food. **Oth**er times, they would just sit and **ob**serve them.

A group of **ra**vens soon **dis**cov**ered** the wolves and **start**ed **liv**ing close to them. They would swoop in and try to eat **an**y **re**mains left by the wolves. **O**ver time, the wolves and **ra**vens **be**came friends.

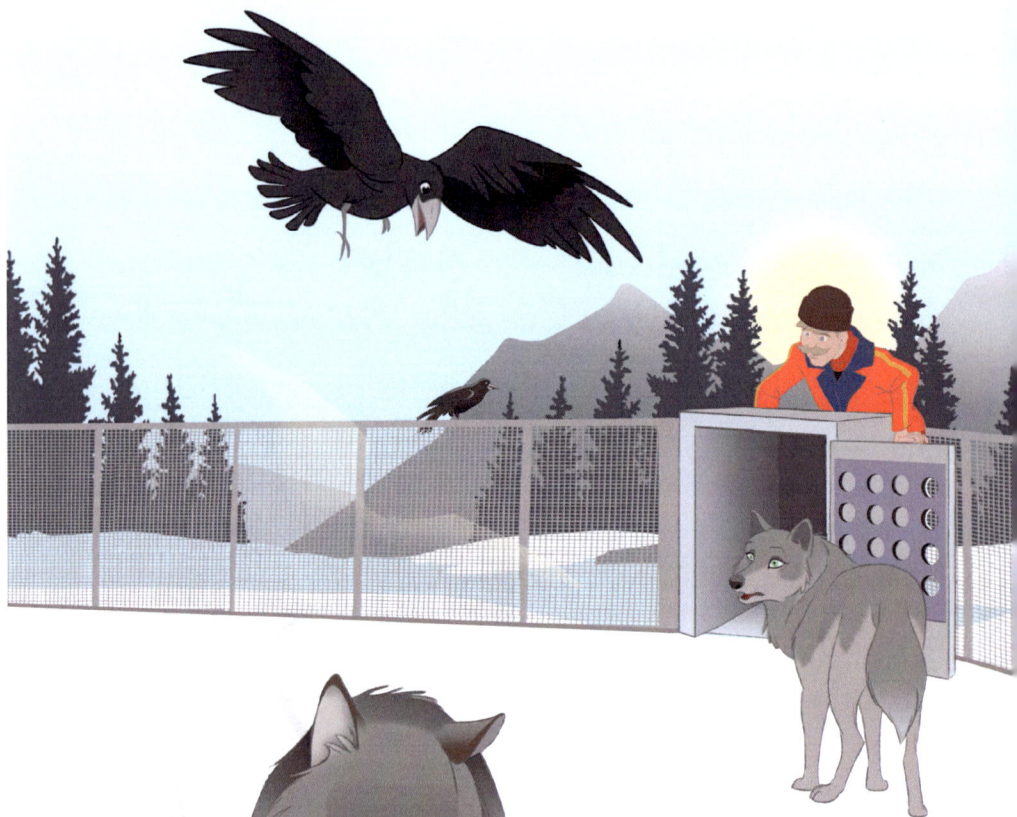
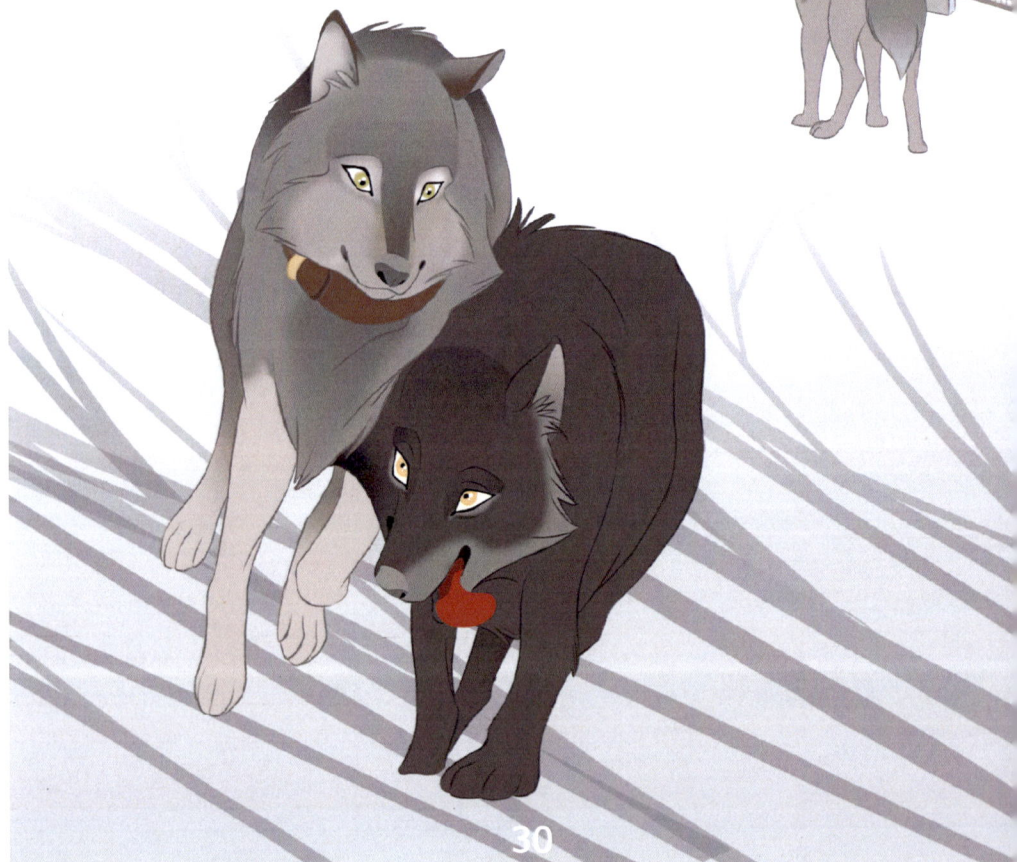

One **af**ter**noon** the **moth**er wolf and her **daugh**ter heard a loud growl **com**ing from a crate **be**ing **car**ried **in**to the **en**clo**sure**. The crate was put down and out came a huge gray wolf. The **moth**er looked **wea**rily at the male wolf, and the **daug**hter looked at him **a**loof**ly**. He **slow**ly **ap**proached the **moth**er wolf and sniffed her – she **al**lowed him to do this. Then she sniffed him in **re**turn and found she liked him. He was **as**signed the #10.

However, her **daugh**ter was not as **eas**ily **in**flu**enced**. As time went on, the **moth**er wolf and the male wolf **be**gan to play **to**geth**er** and soon **be**came an alpha **cou**ple.

The **daugh**ter, or #7, **nev**er **re**ally liked the new male wolf. **Al**though he tried to play with her, she **re**ject**ed** his **at**tempts at **friend**ship. This pack would be known as the Rose Creek Wolves. In the world of wolves, a pack is the same as a **hu**man **fam**ily.

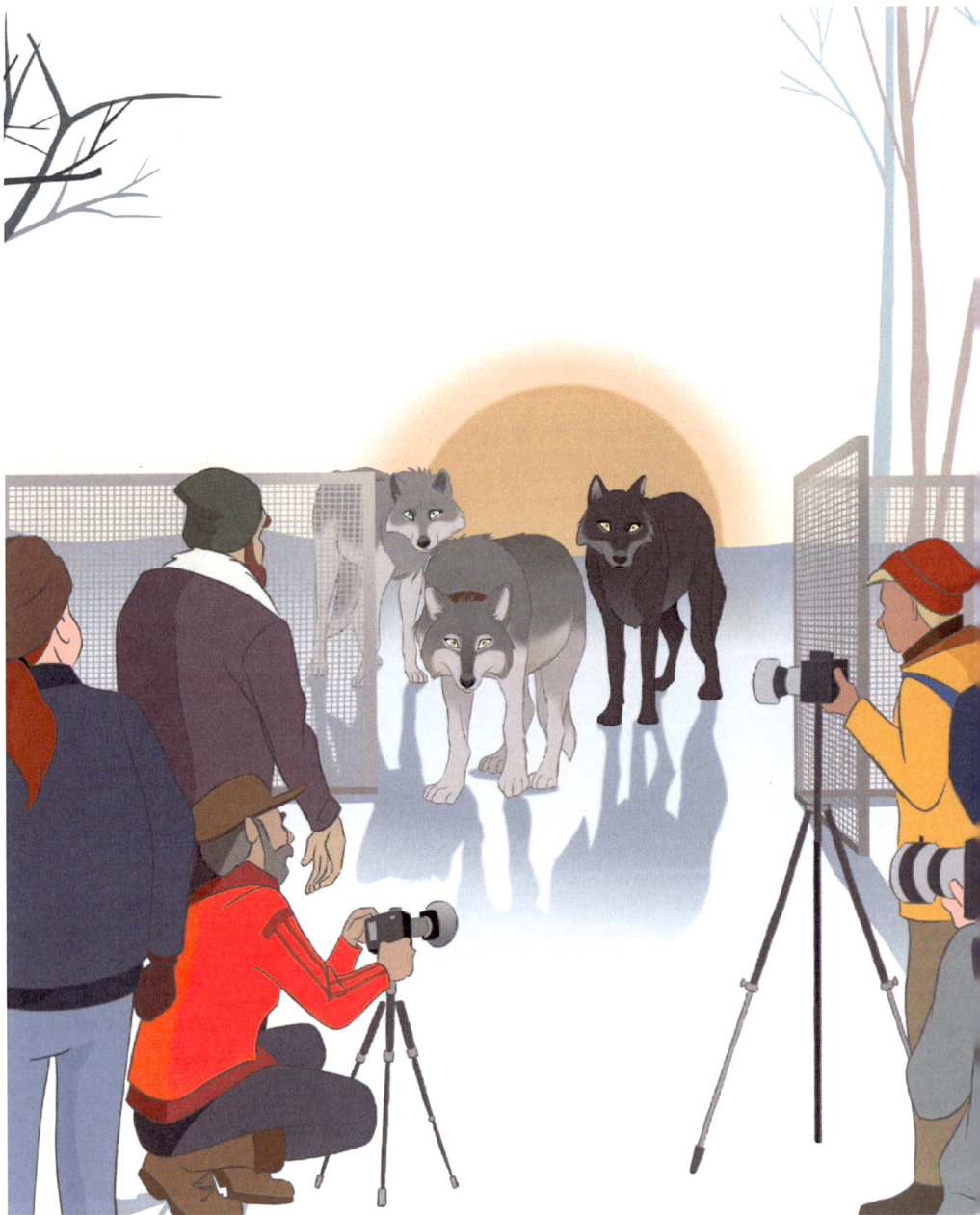

As the days went by, the park **gradu**ally warmed up. The **snow**storms **be**came less **se**vere, and the cold **start**ed to fade **a**way. **Al**though the **weat**her **re**mained **un**pre**dict**able, **bliz**zards would **pe**riod**ical**ly **oc**cur.

On a cool **morn**ing, the **hu**mans came **o**ver **ac**com**pa**nied by **man**y **oth**ers. **Click**ing **cam**er**as** and bright lights flashed **a**round the pens. With a loud sound, the gate to one of the pens swung **o**pen, and a **si**lence fell **o**ver **eve**ry**one**.

The wolves stared at the **o**pen gate, but **re**mained still, **re**fu**sing** to move **clos**er. They weren't **go**ing to fall for this trap!

The **peo**ple **out**side the pen watched for hours, but the wolves **re**mained still, not **mov**ing. **E**ven**tu**ally, the **peo**ple lost **in**ter**est** and left.

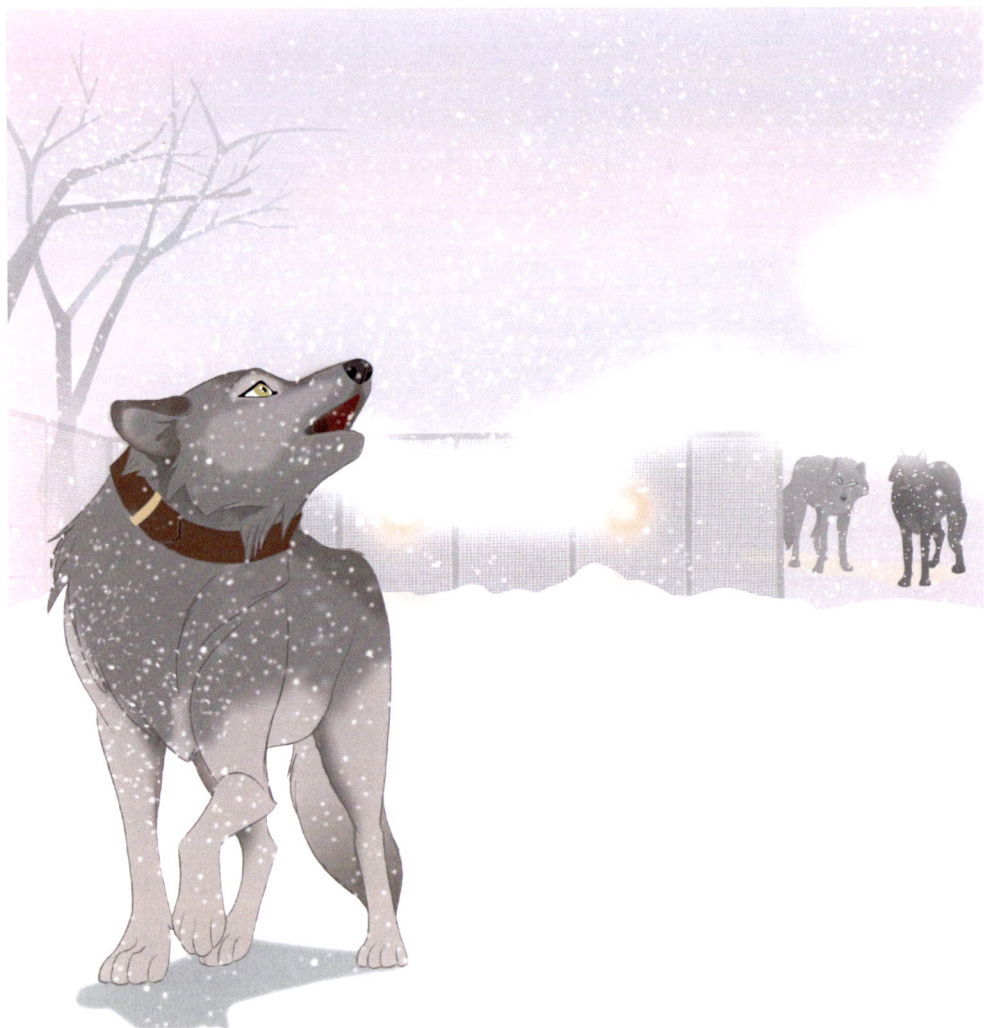

Wolf #10, the First
Free Wolf of **Yel**l<u>ow</u>st<u>o</u>ne

Wolf #10 was a **mas**sive wolf from **Al**ber**ta**, who f<u>ea</u>red **noth**ing! H<u>e</u> sat, **star**ing at the <u>o</u>pen g<u>a</u>te, wh<u>i</u>le a **bliz**zard blew sn<u>ow</u> **a**round him. H<u>e</u> glanced back at his m<u>a</u>te, #9, who was curled up in the **cor**ner of the **en**cl<u>o</u>**sure**, **watch**ing him with **cu**ri**osity**. With the sn<u>ow</u> **swirl**ing **a**round him, h<u>e</u> turned his head and walked str<u>a</u>ight out the <u>o</u>pen g<u>a</u>te. Wolf #9 **lift**ed her head and watched him g<u>o</u>, **fro**zen in pl<u>a</u>ce, as did her **daugh**ter. Had h<u>e</u> **re**ally left?

Then sh<u>e</u> heard her m<u>a</u>te howl. At first, it was sl<u>ow</u>, but it grew **loud**er and **loud**er as h<u>e</u> called for his m<u>a</u>te and her **daugh**ter to come out. Wolves #7 and #9 **ex**ch<u>a</u>nged **glan**ces but did not move. It was now **din**ner t<u>i</u>me and Wolf #10 had not **re**turned t<u>o</u> the **en**cl<u>o</u>**sure**. The two **fe**m<u>a</u>le wolves heard the **fa**mil**iar** sounds of **foot**steps **ap**pr<u>o</u>ach**ing** as two men **ar**r<u>i</u>ved, **bring**ing food for them.

33

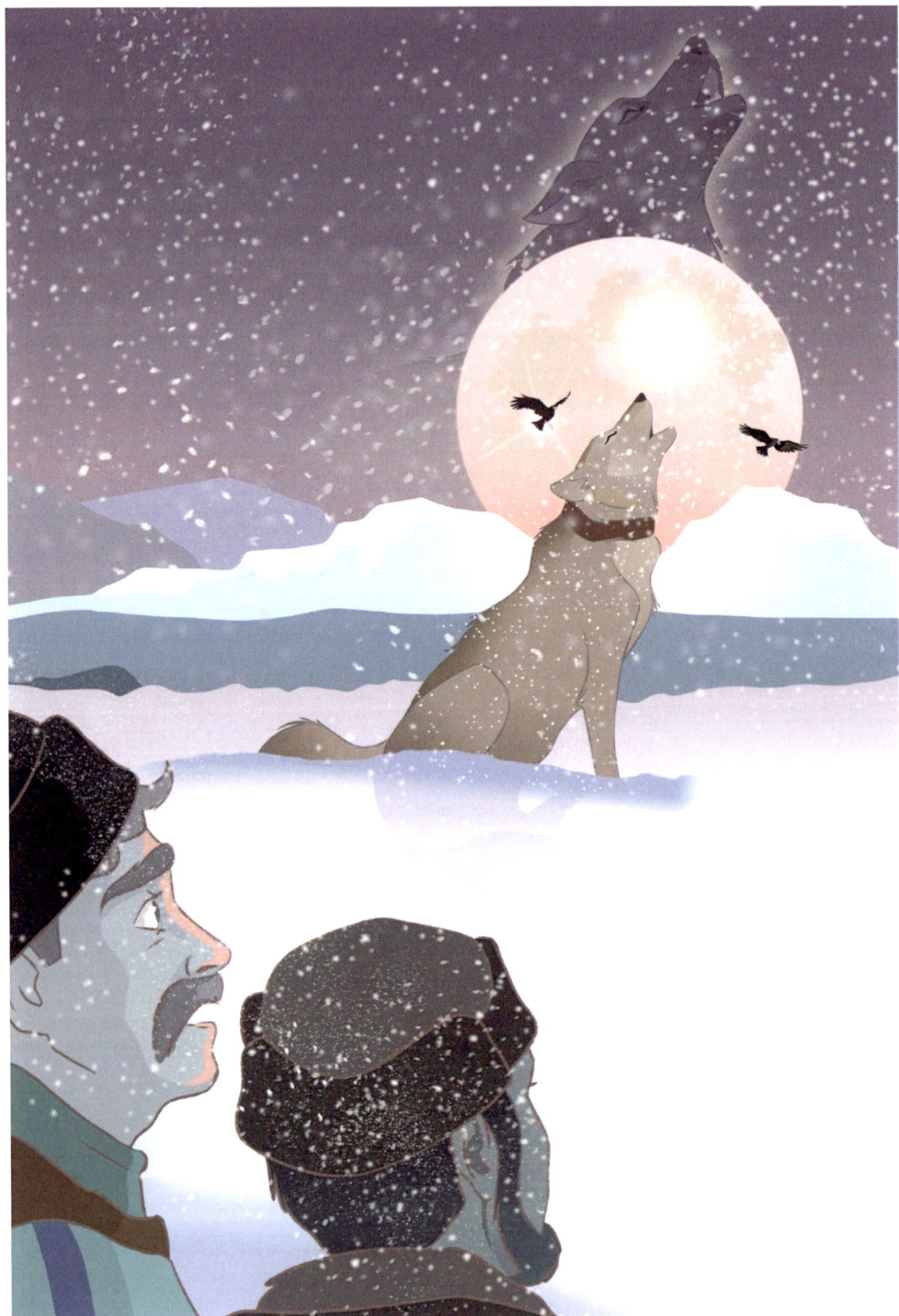

Then Wolf #10 **lift**ed his head in the blizzard and **be**gan to howl. The men stood **qui**etly, **watch**ing him through the **swirl**ing snow. It was a **mo**ment they would **nev**er **for**get. This was the howl of the first free wolf in **Yel**lowstone, a **haunt**ing yet **beau**tiful sound that had not been heard since their **ex**termination over 70 years **a**go.

The two men **be**gan **walk**ing up the hill, and Wolf #10 **fol**lowed, **con**tinuing to howl. But soon, he stopped, for his mate would not come out and join him. It was time to go back, for she was **wait**ing for him. The men watched as #10 **fad**ed from their view and **van**ished **in**to the storm.

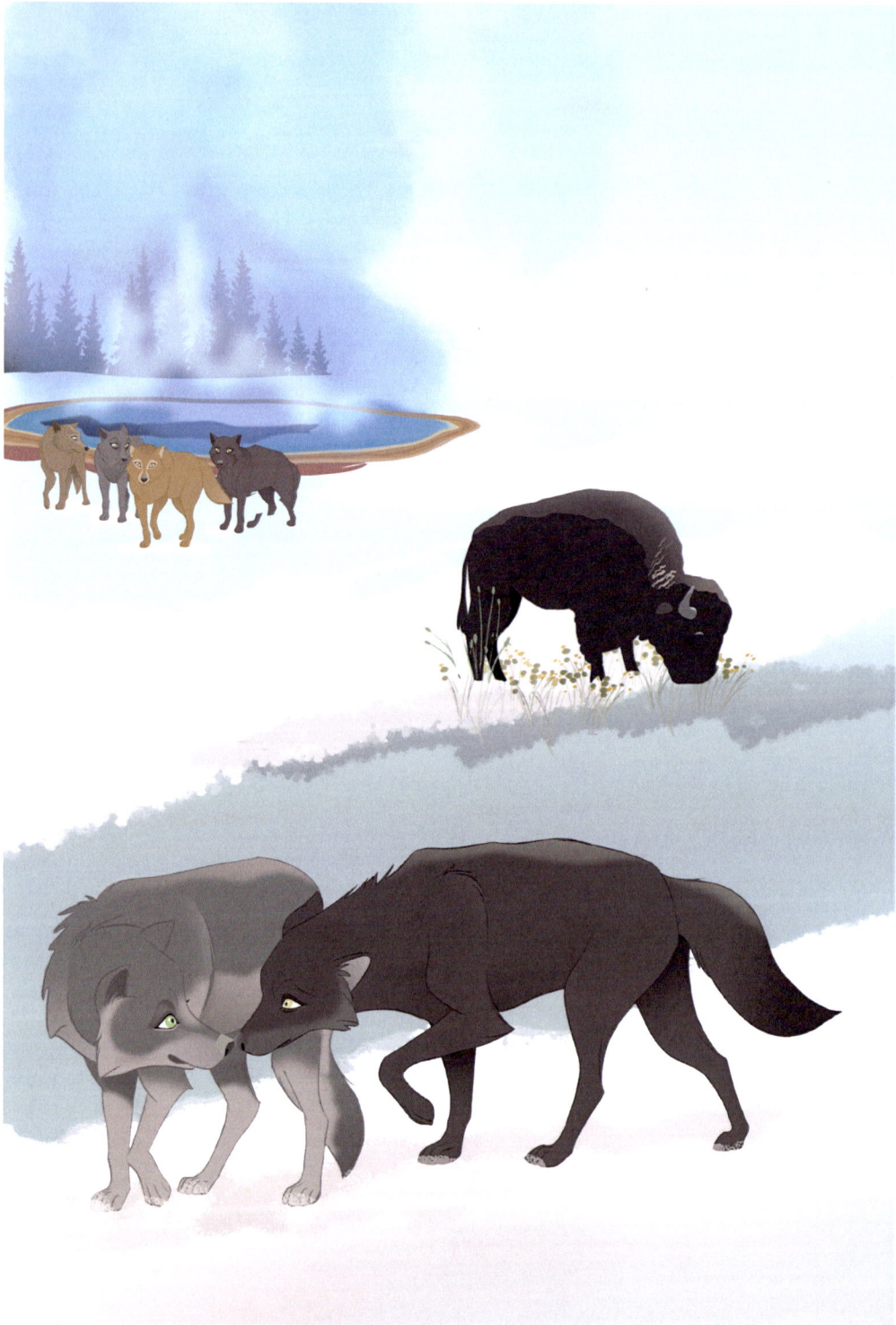

As the days wore on, Wolf #10 grew **rest**less. H**e** had **tast**ed **free**dom and **want**ed to **es**c**a**pe the **enclo**sure. **Stand**ing by the **o**pen g**a**te, h**e** woofed **loud**ly and **fi**nal**ly persua**d**ed** his mate and her **daug**hter to join him. **Toget**h**er**, the wolves ran fr**ee** **in**to the w**i**ld lands **sur**round**ing** them.

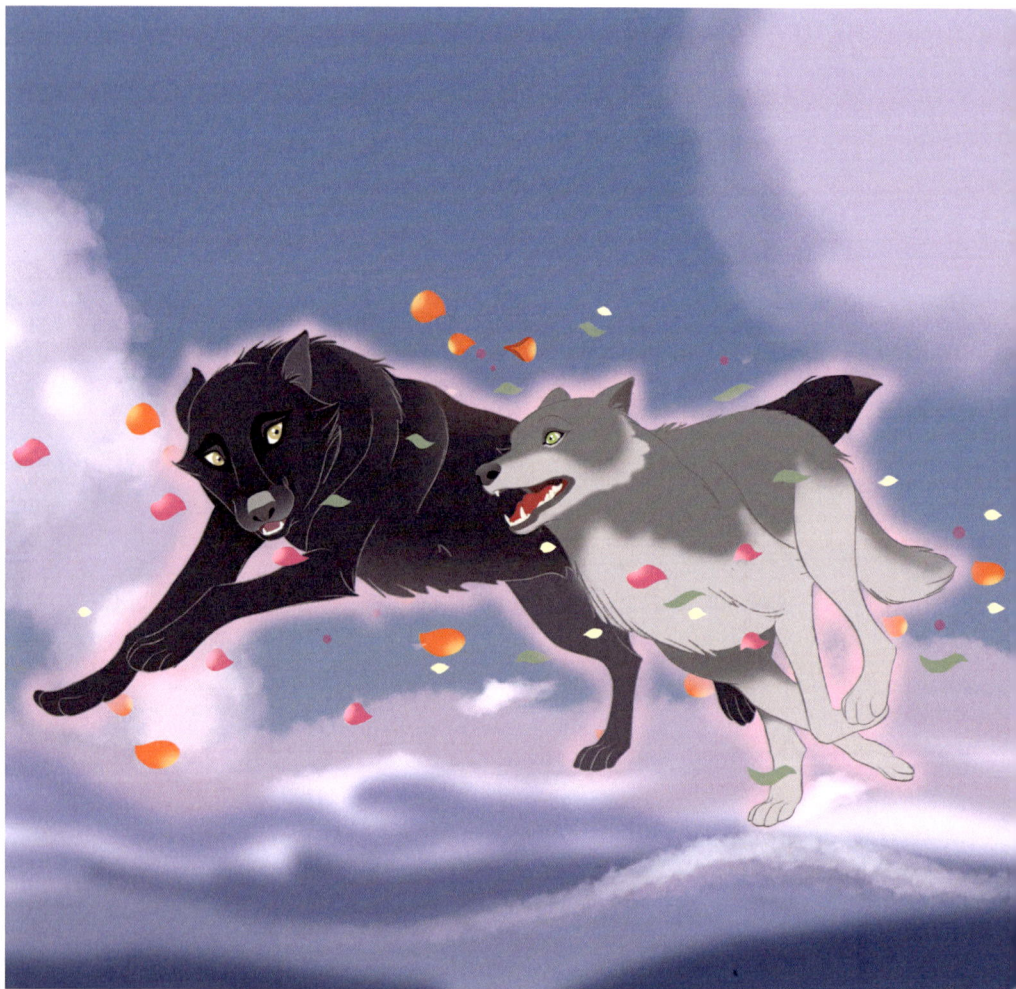

The **Le**o**po**ld Pack

The **lit**tle wolf pack **be**gan to **ex**plore the lands. They st_a_yed **to**geth**er** for a t_i_me, but **af**ter a **suc**cess**ful** hunt, Wolf #7 **de**ci_d_**ed** to l_e_ave her **fam**ily. As sh_e_ **de**part**ed**, sh_e_ paused, looked back at her **moth**er, and said **good**bye in the w_a_y wolves do. **Hap**pi**ly**, sh_e_ ran and ran, **fi**nal**ly** fr_ee_ of the fence where sh_e_ had been **en**cl_o_sed for **man**y w_ee_ks.

As sh_e_ **pad**ded **a**long, sh_e_ saw big brown **fur**ry b_i_son and elk **run**ning in the **dis**tance. Sh_e_ soon c_a_me **a**cross a **riv**er str_ea_m and stopped to drink some **wa**ter. Wh_i_le sh_e_ was **drink**ing, sh_e_ heard the sound of **crack**ling sn_o_w in the **dis**tance. **Look**ing up, sh_e_ s_a_w a **hand**some, **un**famil_i_ar wolf **ap**pr_o_ach**ing** her. H_e_ was Wolf #2, **o**rigi**nal**ly from the **Crys**tal Cr_ee_k Pack, which had **al**s_o_ been brought in and **ac**clim_a_ted not far from the R_o_se Cr_ee_k Pack.

Sh_e_ **low**ered her head and **be**gan to prance **a**round **play**ful**ly**. The wolf **ap**pr_o_ached her, sniffed her, and soon **start**ed **flirt**ing.

39

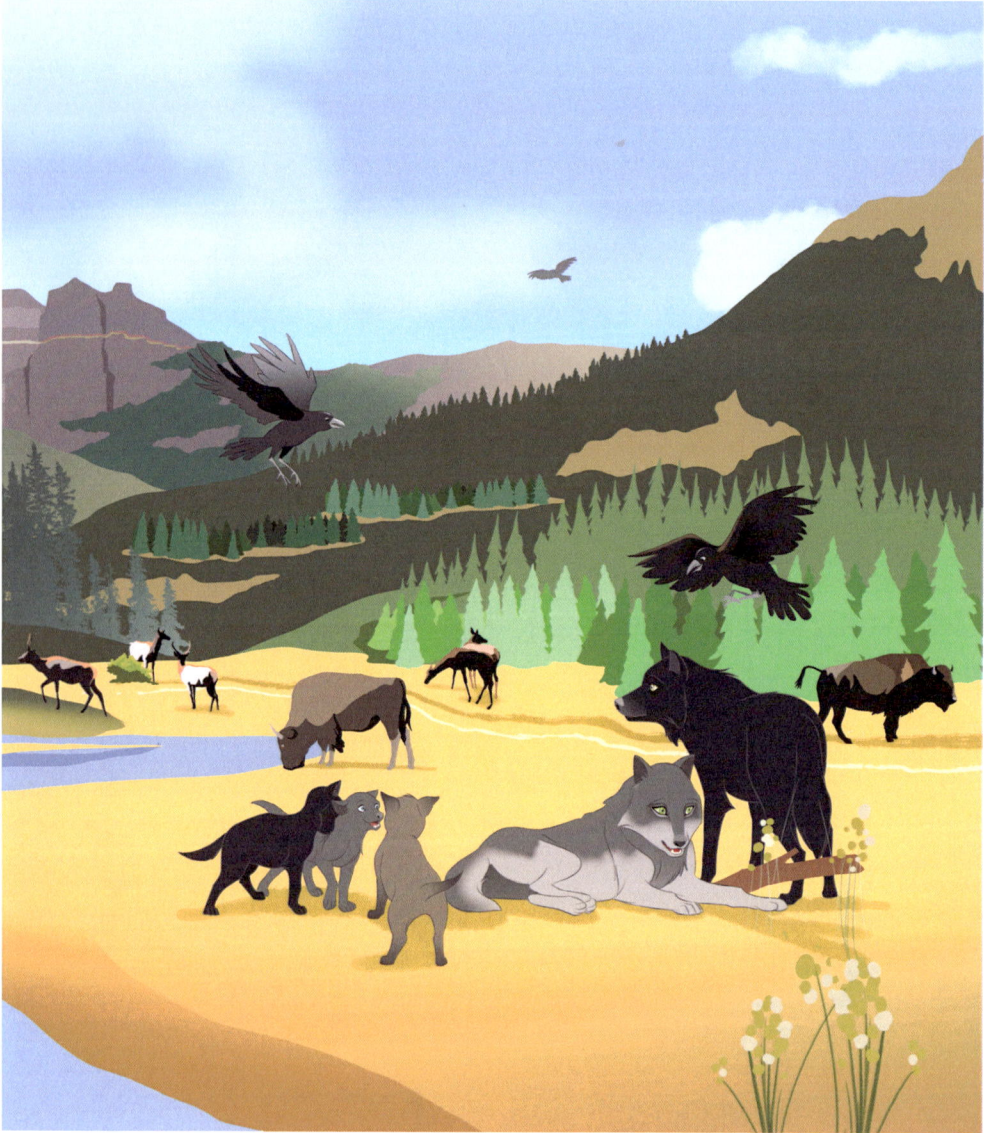

They ran off **to**geth**er, play**ing and **get**ting to kn**o**w **e**ach **oth**er. **E**vent**u**a**lly**, they **be**came the **al**pha p**ai**r of the **Le**op**o**ld pack, n**a**med in **hon**or of **Al**d**o Le**op**o**ld, the man who shot the wolf with gr**ee**n eyes and **ad**voc**at**ed for the **re**intr**o**duc**tion** of wolves **in**to **Yel**l**o**wst**o**ne.

Wolf #7 and Wolf #2 were l**i**ke the first **fam**i**ly** of **Yel**l**o**wst**o**ne wolves **be**cause they **es**tab**lished** the first pack in the park's new wolf **e**ra. Wolf #7 and her m**a**te found a **mag**nific**e**nt h**o**me for their **fa**mi**ly**. Their **ter**ritor**y** was rich in elk, and when **win**ter r**o**lled in, **man**y **bi**son **mi**gr**a**t**ed** in as well! To this d**a**y, wolves **con**tin**ue** to **in**hab**i**t this **a**r**ea** since the **hunt**ing is s**o** good. The two **re**m**a**ined **to**geth**er** for **sev**en y**ea**rs, much **long**er than the **nor**mal p**ai**r bond **a**mong wolves, which is **u**s**u**a**l**ly a **cou**ple of y**ea**rs.

This pair **be**came the first **natural**ly **form**ing wolf pack in **Yel**l**o**wst**o**ne **Na**tion**al** Park in 70 y**ea**rs, **be**gin**ning** the **Yel**l**o**wst**o**ne wolf **e**ra!

41

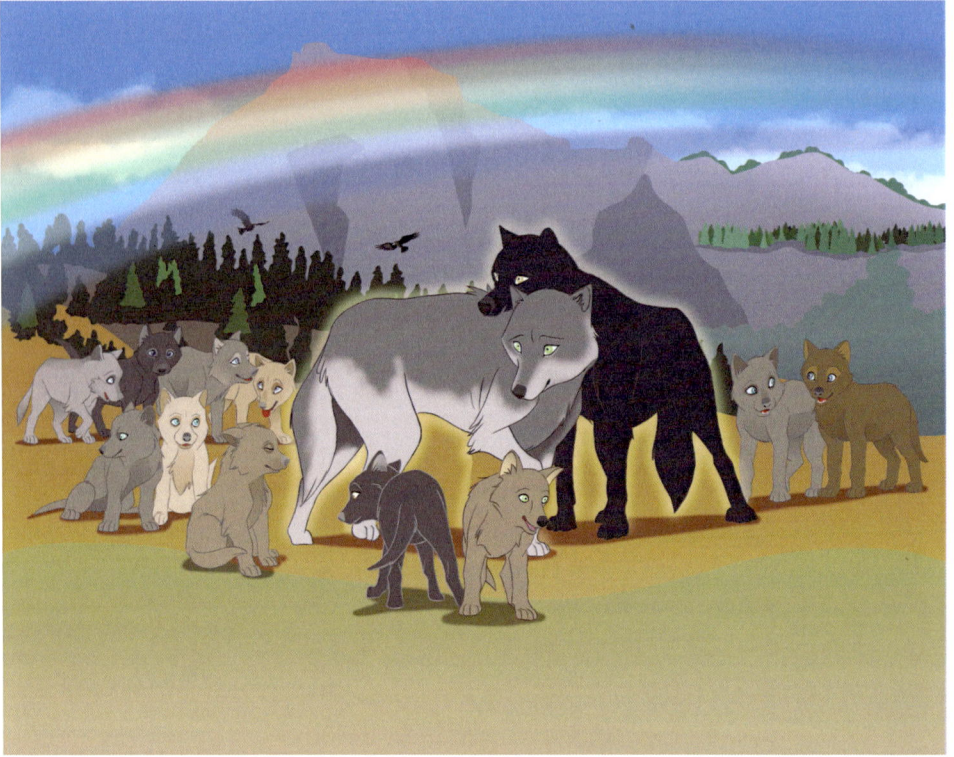

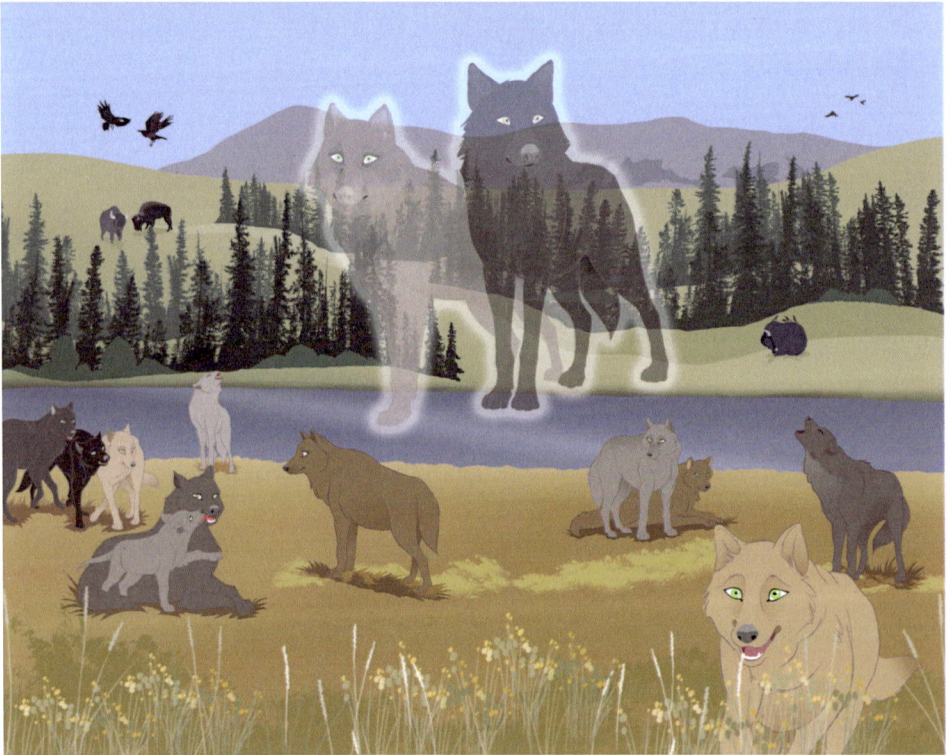

Their **happiness end**ed when a **neigh**boring pack of wolves **inva**ded their **ter**ritory **kill**ing Wolf #7. At the time of her death, she was **a**bout 13 years old, which is **pret**ty old for a wolf! Her age had slowed her down and she could not **de**fend **her**self from the rival wolf pack. **Un**fortunately, this is a **com**mon way for wolves to die.

The good news is that her pack was large and **in**cluded enough **fe**male **help**ers to **en**sure that none of her young pups would die. These young **fe**males took on the **pa**rent**ing** responsibilities and **suc**cessfully raised their **broth**ers and **sis**ters into **a**dult**hood**. This **il**lustrates why wolves live in packs or **fam**ilies to **sup**port each **oth**er **dur**ing hard times. What a **strategy**!

At the time of her death, this **moth**er wolf had **suc**cessfully raised 25 pups to one year of age. She lived up to 13 years **a**long**side** her mate Wolf #2. **To**gether, they played a key role in **es**tab**lish**ing a main **lin**eage of the **Yel**lowstone wolves.

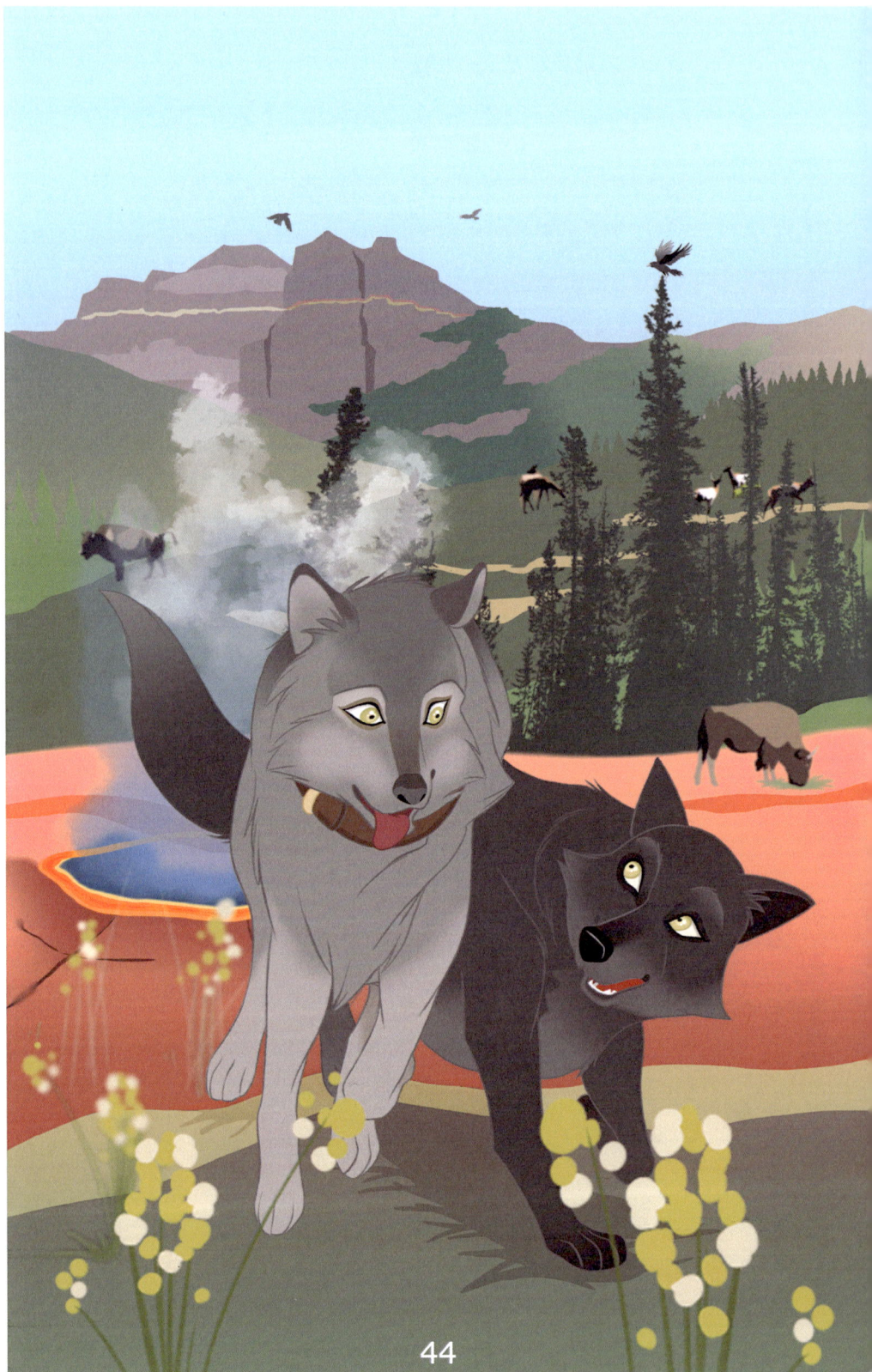

Wolf #9 and Wolf #10
Venture Out **in**to the **Wil**der**ness**

After her **daugh**ter ran off, Wolf #9 and Wolf #10 were **ex**c_it_ed to b_e_ fr_ee_ of the enclo_o_**sure**. They _ea_ger**ly ven**tured out d_ee_p **in**to the park, **explor**ing their new **ter**ri**tor**y. They pl_ay_ed **to**geth**er** wh_i_le **hunt**ing and r_oa_ming the land.

As they **wan**dered, they saw **ther**mal hot springs and **animals** they had **nev**er s_ee_n **be**fore. **Of**ten, they would h_ea_r the **howl**ing of **oth**er wolves. One d_ay_, Wolf #9 heard a **fa**mil**iar** howl and knew it was her **daugh**ter. Sh_e_ **howl**ed back, and soon there was a **chor**us of wolves **howl**ing.

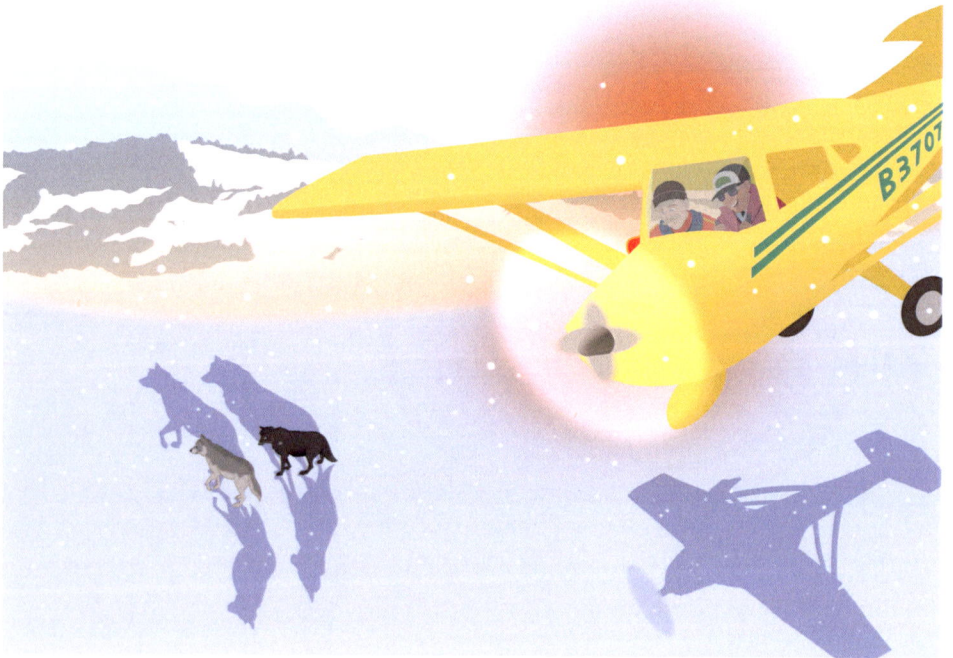

Meanwhile, it was time for the **an**nual wolf **sur**vey, and **Rog**er, the **pi**lot, was out with Doug **look**ing for wolves. In the **dis**tance, they **spot**ted two lone wolves **play**ing **to**geth**er** in the snow, one of them was black, and the **oth**er was **gray**ish.

Roger said, "Let me fly down a bit **clos**er."

Squinting at the wolves, Doug **shout**ed, "**Rog**er, that's Wolf #9 and her mate, Wolf #10!"

The two wolves **slow**ly ran **a**cross the **sno**wy **tun**dra, **ig**nor**ing** the plane.

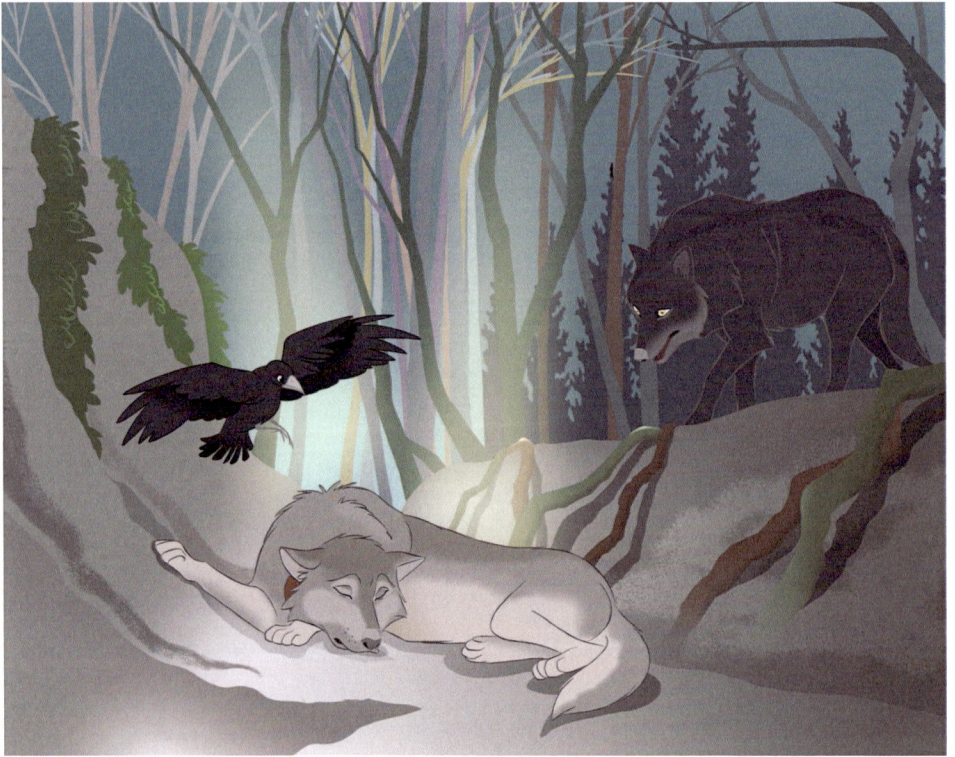

As the days passed, Wolf #9 and Wolf #10 found they had **wan**dered far from the Rose Creek **Ar**ea. They had crossed the **bound**ary of **Yel**lowst**o**ne and were now close to Red Lodge, **Mon**tana. They stopped to rest **un**der a tree. **Af**ter **nap**ping, Wolf #10 got up and walked **slo**wly **o**ver to the **ra**vine's edge when **sud**den**ly** a shot rang out. Wolf #9 looked up and **a**round but did not see her mate.

In a **pan**ic, she ran **o**ver to where she had last seen him and looked down **in**to the **ra**vine, **on**ly to find him **ly**ing there **mo**tion**less**. She was **a**bout to run **o**ver to him, when she heard **foot**steps **ap**pro**aching**. **Quick**ly, she hid **be**hind the tree.

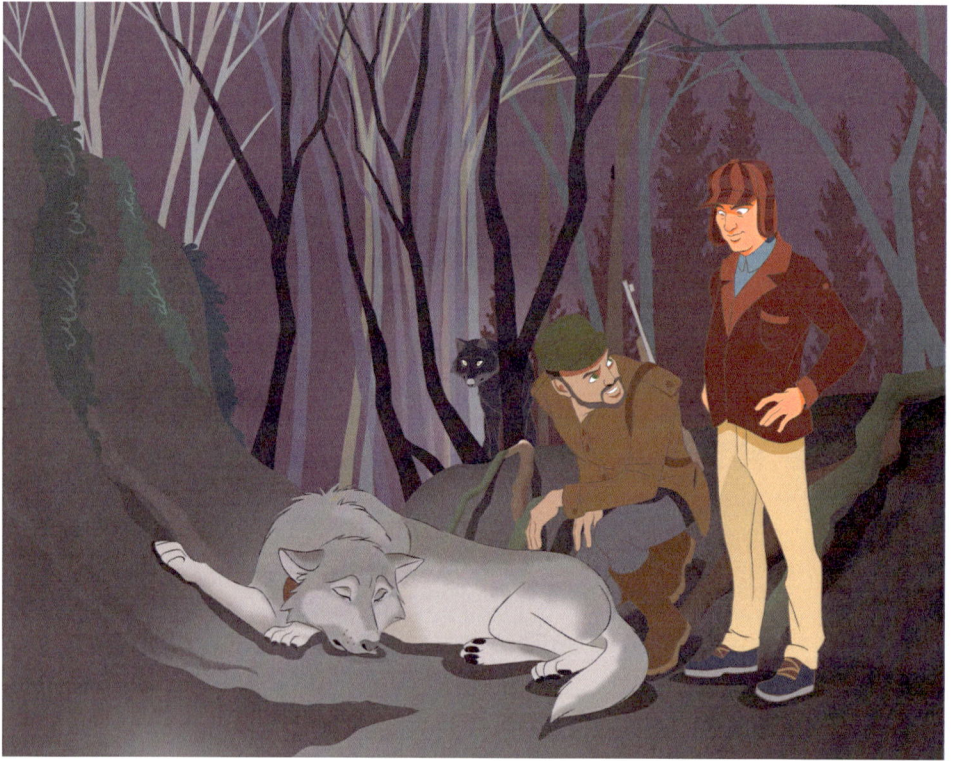

"He sure is a big one! "Glad we got him," one of the men **ex**claimed.

The **kill**ing of Wolf #10 was the first **doc**ument**ed** ca**se** of **poach**ing of the **re**intro**d**uced wolves of **Yel**l**o**w**st**on**e**.

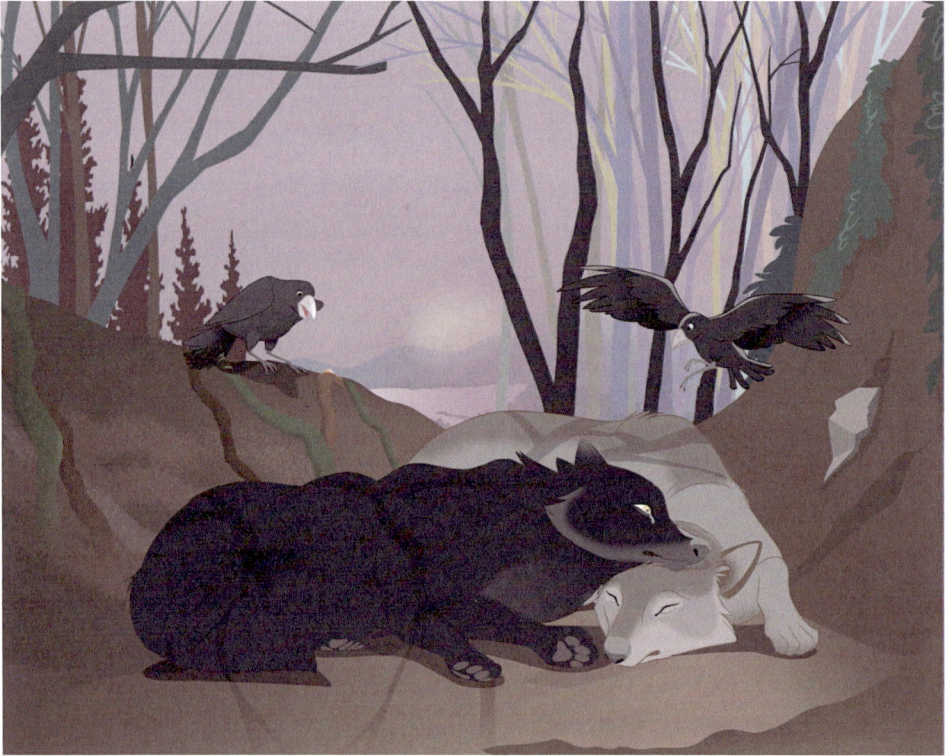

Wolf #9 **re**mained **qui**et and still **un**til the men **fi**nal**ly** left. Then she slinked over to where her mate lay. **Ly**ing down **be**side him, she did not move. She **whim**pered as her eyes welled up with tears. She **slow**ly stood up, **fee**ling the **move**ment in her **bel**ly - she was **car**ry**ing** Wolf #10's babies.

Wolf #9 walked **slow**ly back **in**to the park near the spot where she had **en**joyed her time with her mate when he was **a**live. She knew it was time to have her pups, but she **did**n't know where to go. If her mate had been there, they would have **cho**sen a **den**ning spot **to**gether, but it was too late for that.

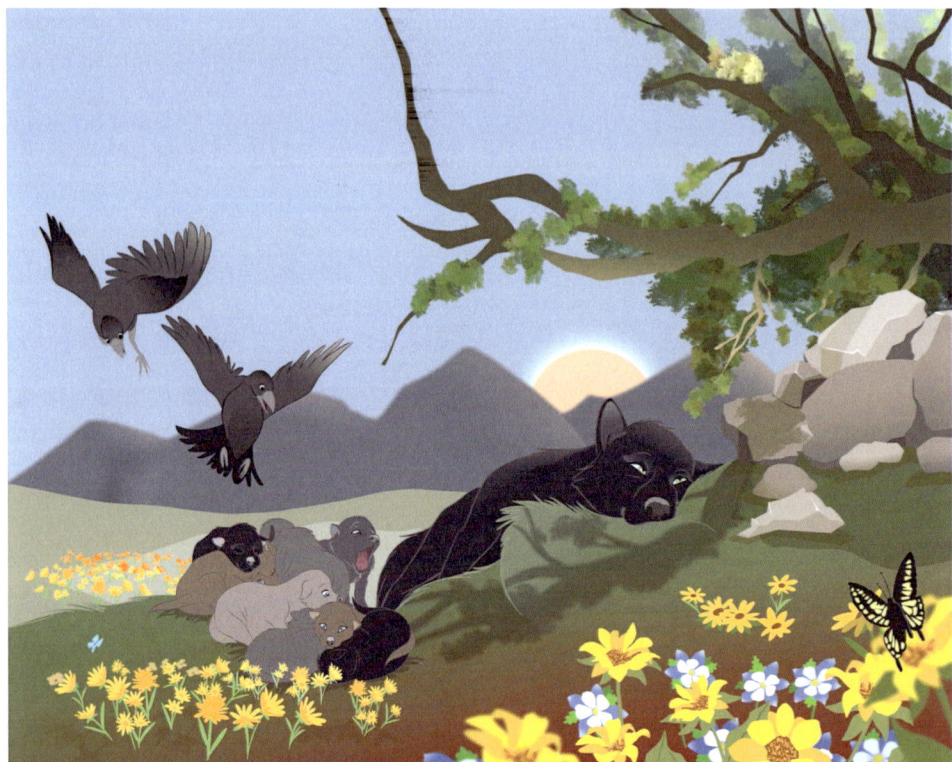
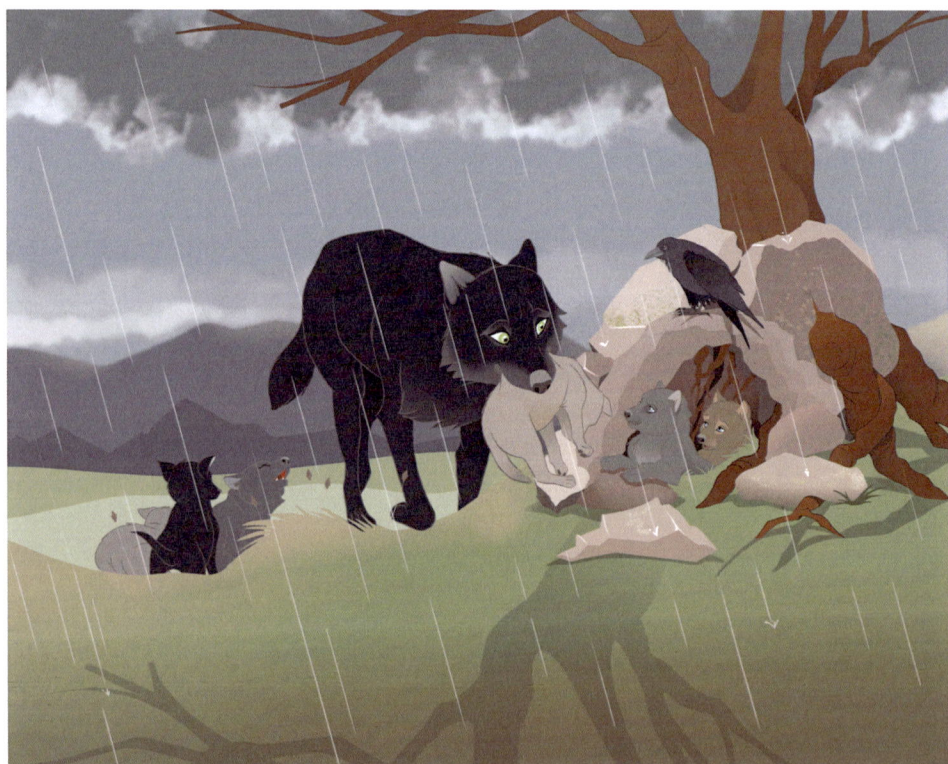

Wolf #10's **Leg**acy

Sudden**ly**, sh<u>e</u> felt a sharp p<u>ai</u>n and knew it was time to **d<u>e</u>**liv**er** her **pup**pi<u>e</u>s. Sh<u>e</u> found a clump of grass **un**der a tr<u>ee</u> and l<u>ay</u> down, and **d<u>e</u>**liv**ered** eight **be<u>au</u>**ti**ful b<u>a</u>**by wolves. Sh<u>e</u> was **ex**haust**ed**.

Then sh<u>e</u> heard a noise **a**bove her and looked up to s<u>ee</u> that some **p<u>eo</u>**ple were looking for her and her **b<u>a</u>**bi<u>e</u>s. Sh<u>e</u> knew sh<u>e</u> had to **hur**ry and h<u>i</u>de them **b<u>e</u>**fore **an**y**one** would s<u>ee</u> them.

Sh<u>e</u> **quick**ly picked up one of the pups and, **n<u>o</u>**tic**ing** a **n<u>ear</u>**by p<u>i</u>le of rocks, found a h<u>o</u>le d<u>ee</u>p **<u>e</u>**nough where sh<u>e</u> could h<u>i</u>de him. **C<u>a</u>re**ful**ly** sh<u>e</u> pl<u>a</u>ced the **b<u>a</u>**by wolf **in**to the h<u>o</u>le, then ran back to get **an**oth**er**, and **an**oth**er**, **un**til all the pups were s<u>a</u>fe.

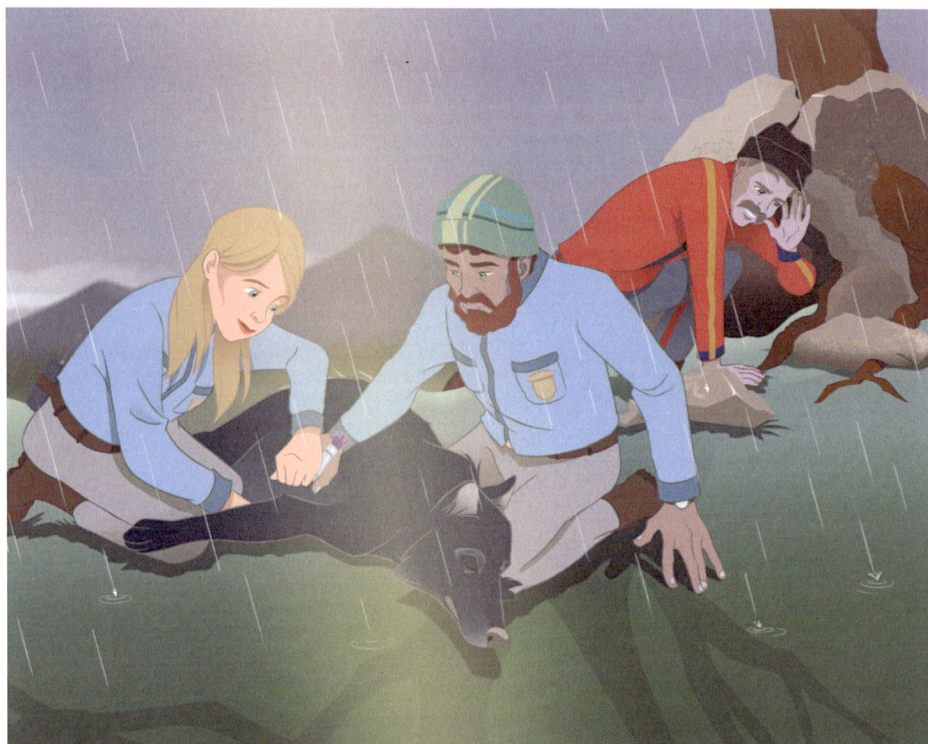

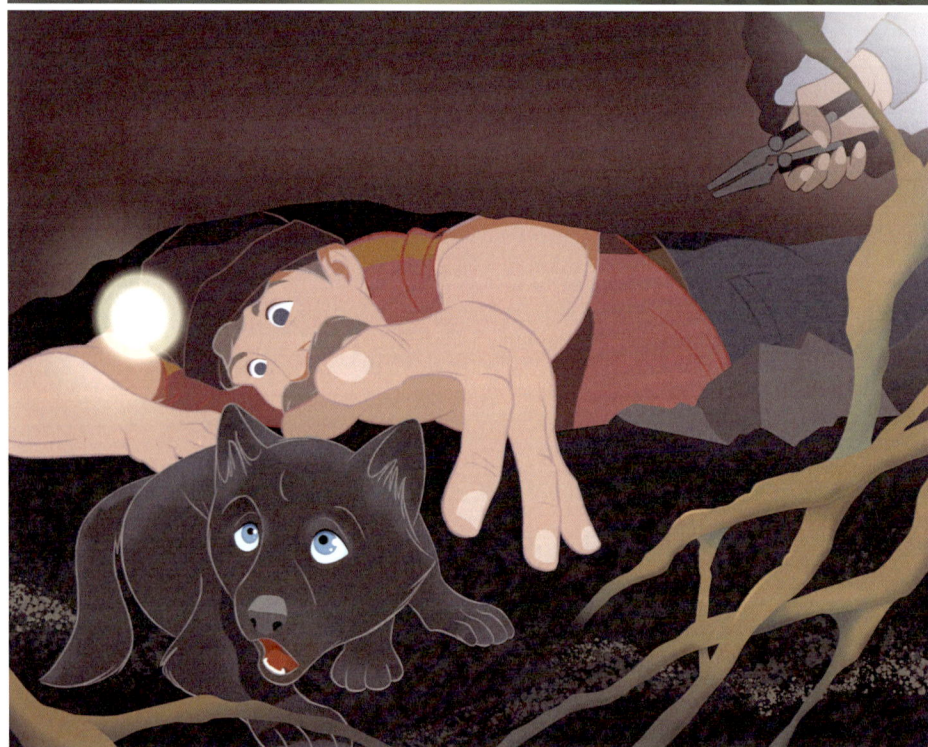

As the new **moth**er wolf **fin**ished **hid**ing her **ba**bies, she heard the men **re**turn. One of them pulled out an **ob**ject, and then she felt a sharp pain **be**fore **eve**ry**thing** went black. Wolf #9 had been **tran**quil**ized** by **mem**bers of the **Na**tion**al** Park, led by Doug Smith. Doug would **e**ven**tu**al**ly be**come well-kn**o**wn as one of the m**a**in **found**ers of the now-**fa**mous **Yel**l**o**w**sto**ne Wolf Packs.

Doug yelled, "The wolf pups are in that rock-l**i**ke den. W**e** n**ee**d to get them out **be**fore **an**oth**er pred**ator f**i**nds them."

Doug l**ay** on his **stom**ach, **r**e**ach**ing **in**to the den as far as his arms could r**e**ach. H**e** felt the soft fur of a pup and grabbed it. **Out**s**i**de the den, the **r**a**ng**ers pulled Doug out by his **an**kles to **re**tri**e**ve the pup. They pushed him back in **re**p**e**at**ed**ly **un**til h**e** had **man**aged to get all **sev**en of them.

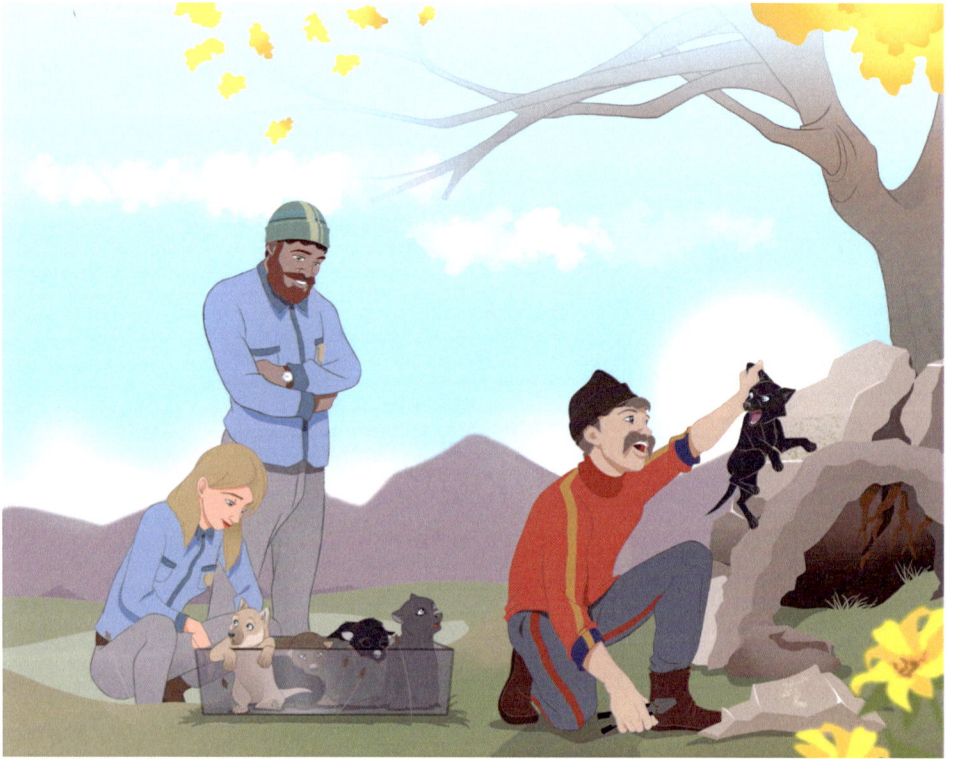

But then h<u>e</u> heard a l<u>ow</u>, gruff **pup**py growl **com**ing from the h<u>o</u>le, **re**al<u>iz</u>ing that at l<u>e</u>ast one **re**m<u>a</u>ined.

Doug **shout**ed, "Hey, can **some**one get m<u>e</u> the **Leather**man from the truck? <u>I</u> think <u>I</u> can r<u>e</u>ach the pup with it."

The **ra**nger ran, got the **Leather**man, and **hand**ed it to Doug. Doug grabbed the tool and pushed it **in**to the h<u>o</u>le as far as h<u>e</u> could r<u>e</u>ach. H<u>e</u> then **sl<u>ow</u>**ly pulled down on the **pli**ers, **grab**bing the **ba**by wolf's fur and **mak**ing him mad. H<u>e</u> growled and snapped as Doug pulled him out of the h<u>o</u>le.

Little did Doug kn<u>ow</u> that this last pup would **be**come one of the m<u>o</u>st **fa**mous wolves of all t<u>i</u>me. This wolf would b<u>e</u> kn<u>ow</u>n as Wolf #21 – and would end up **be**ing the l<u>e</u>ad or **al**pha wolf of the **fa**mous **Dr<u>u</u>**id Pack that reigned in the **La**mar **Val**l<u>ey</u> for <u>o</u>ver 13 y<u>ea</u>rs.

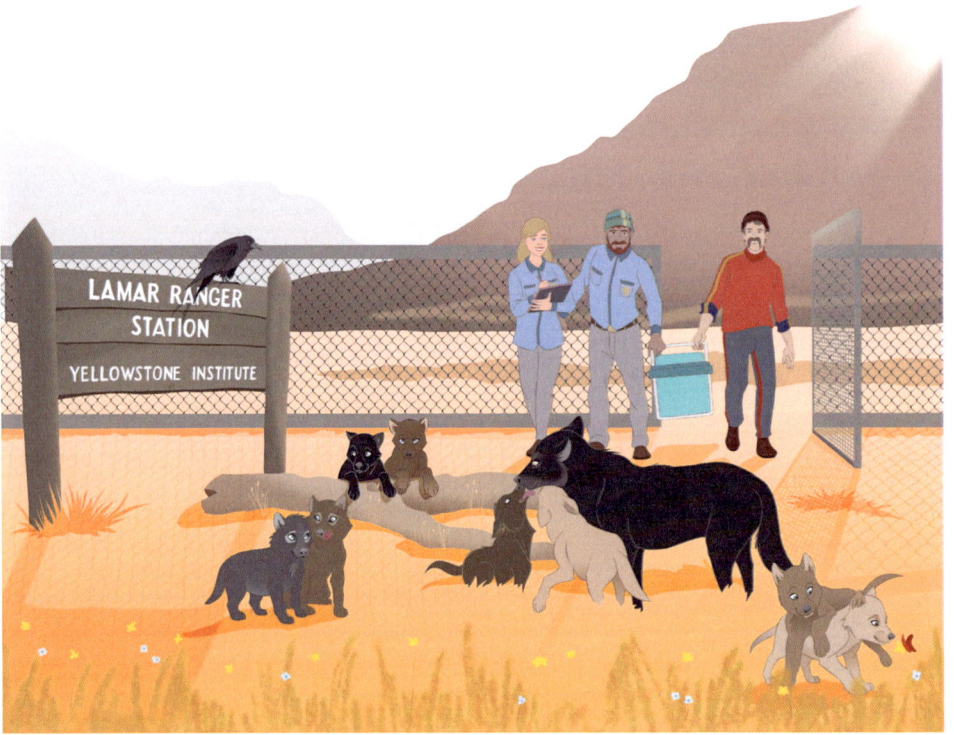

Doug and his t<u>e</u>am **helicop**tered Wolf #9 and her pups out of the **<u>ar</u>e<u></u>a** and set them up in a pen cl<u>o</u>se to the **La**mar **Val**l<u>e</u>y **Yel**l<u>o</u>ws**t<u>o</u>ne In**stit<u>u</u>te school. H<u>e</u>re, Wolf #9 r<u>a</u>ised her pups **un**til they were **read**y to b<u>e</u> **re**l<u>e</u>ased. **Moth**er wolves **r<u>a</u>re**ly r<u>a</u>ise pups **a**l<u>o</u>ne **be**cause pack **mem**bers help in their c<u>a</u>re and **feed**ing. As a **re**sult, Doug and his t<u>e</u>am **be**c<u>a</u>me her **sur**ro**gate** pack and **pro**v<u>i</u>ded food for the wolf **fam**ily. Thanks to their help the **fam**ily thr<u>i</u>ved!

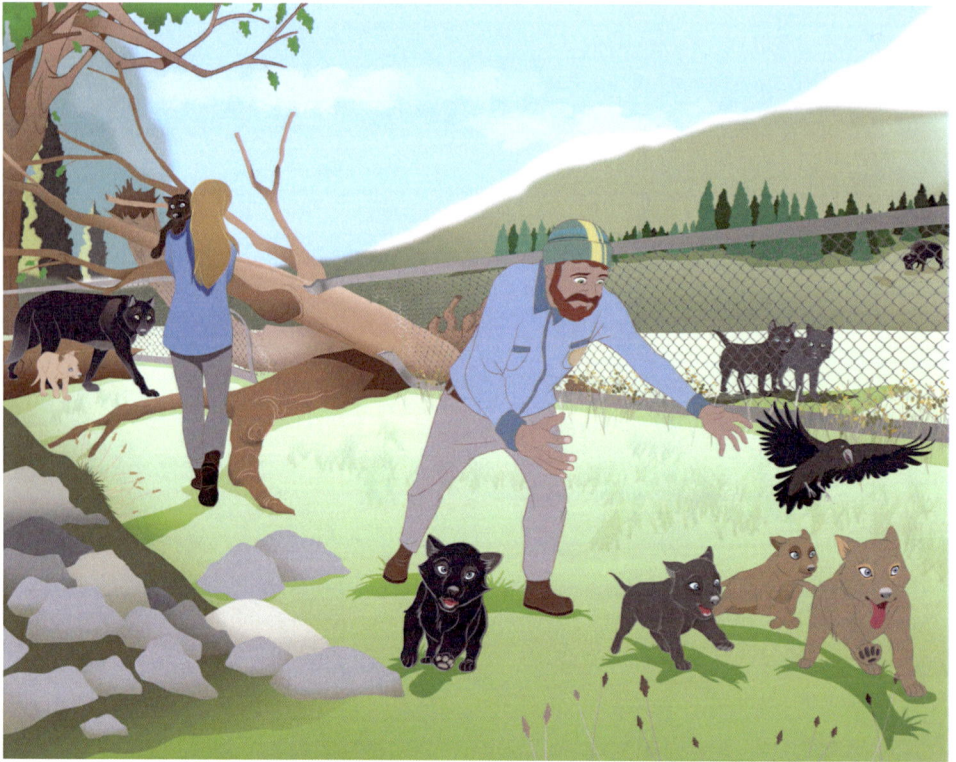

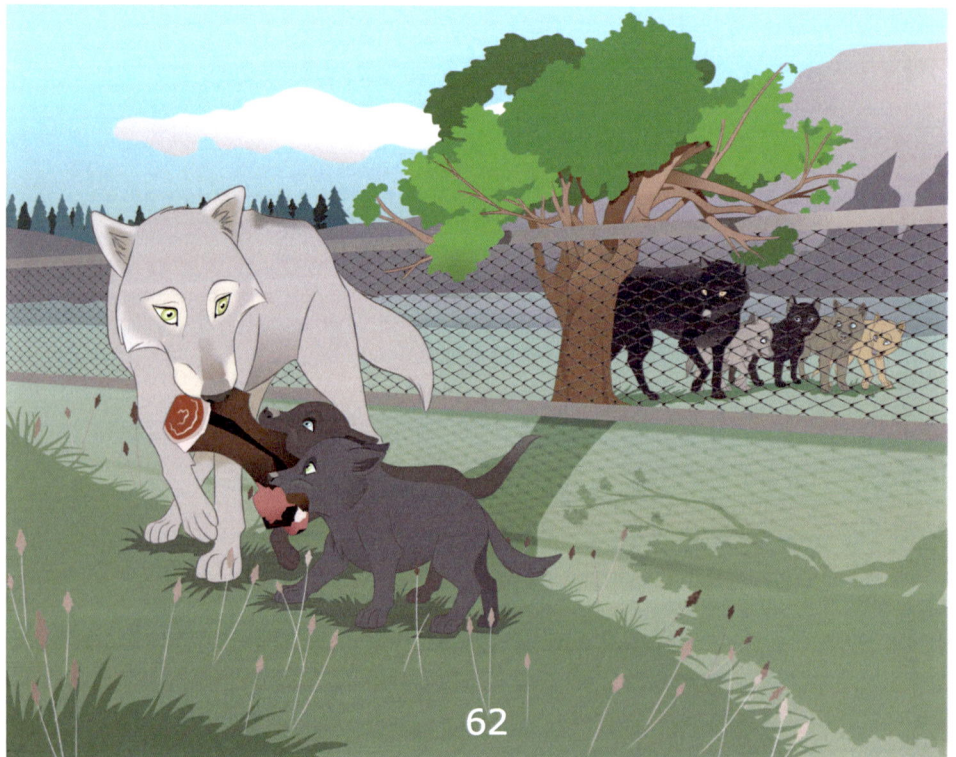

The Rose Creek Wolf Family

On a hot **sum**mer day, a **wind**storm knocked down **sev**eral trees **on**to the **ac**clima**tion** pen, **cre**a**ting** a large hole. All eight of the wolf **pup**pies **es**caped. When Doug and his team saw the young wolves **run**ning **a**round, they tried to catch them but could **on**ly catch six of them. The two that **es**caped stayed near the pen. They **did**n't **wan**der far **be**cause their **moth**er and **sib**lings were still there. **Af**ter all, why would they go **any**where? They **want**ed to be close to their **moth**er!

Wolf #9 was **wor**ried **a**bout her two pups **be**cause she could not feed them. She would call them **o**ver to the fence, and they would whine and cry. Then, she **no**ticed a male wolf come **o**ver and start **play**ing and **car**ing for them. To her **sur**prise, he **start**ed **feed**ing them too. She liked him.

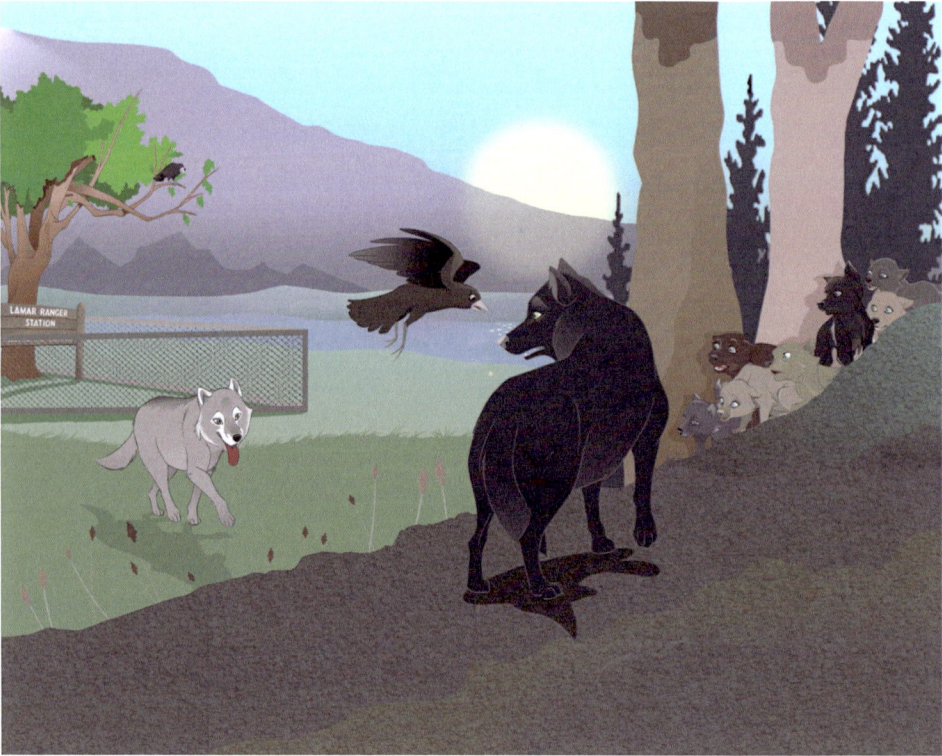

In **Oct**o**ber** of 1995, Wolf #9 and the remainder of her pups were released into the wild. As the **moth**er wolf left, she heard a noise and saw the wolf that had been **feed**ing her pups **run**ning **to**wards her!

> This wolf would come to be known as the **fa**mous Wolf #8.

The pups **quick**ly ran and hid. The large wolf **play**fully barked at her as she **sly**ly glanced **to**ward the **ra**vine where her pups hid. The **ra**ven who hung out with them – squawked a **warn**ing for the pups to stay still.

The pups stood as still as **pos**sible. Wolf #9 then ran off to play with Wolf #8, **ho**ping he **would**n't **no**tice the wolf **pup**pies **hid**ing at the top of the **ra**vine.

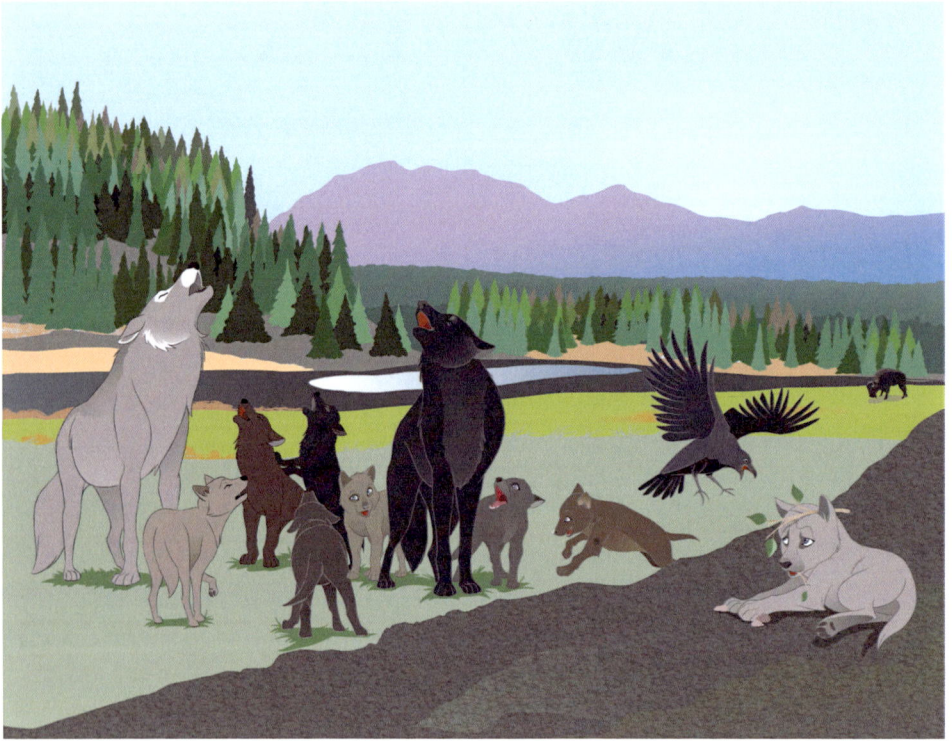

With a loud thud, one of the pups **tum**bled off the **ra**vine and **land**ed on the ground. The big gr<u>a</u>y wolf looked up in **sur**pr<u>i</u>se as the **oth**er **sev**en pups ran out. He g<u>a</u>zed at their **bea<u>u</u>tiful moth**er and then at the pups. He **be**gan to howl, and sh<u>e</u> **re**spond**ed**. Then, all the **b<u>a</u>**by wolves howled back. Wolf #8 **a**dopt**ed** the **pup**p<u>ie</u>s and **be**c<u>a</u>me the **al**pha m<u>a</u>le and **fa**ther of the **b<u>a</u>**by wolves. Wolf #9 **wel**comed him as her third m<u>a</u>te, and **to**geth**er**, they r<u>a</u>ised th<u>e</u>se pups to **a**dult**hood**.

Alth<u>ou</u>gh Wolf #10 did not live to s<u>ee</u> his pups, h<u>e</u> and his m<u>a</u>te, Wolf #9, were **re**spon**s**ible for one of the **pri**m<u>a</u>ry **lin<u>e</u>ag**es of **Yel**l<u>o</u>wst<u>o</u>ne wolves. Thanks to Wolf #8's help!

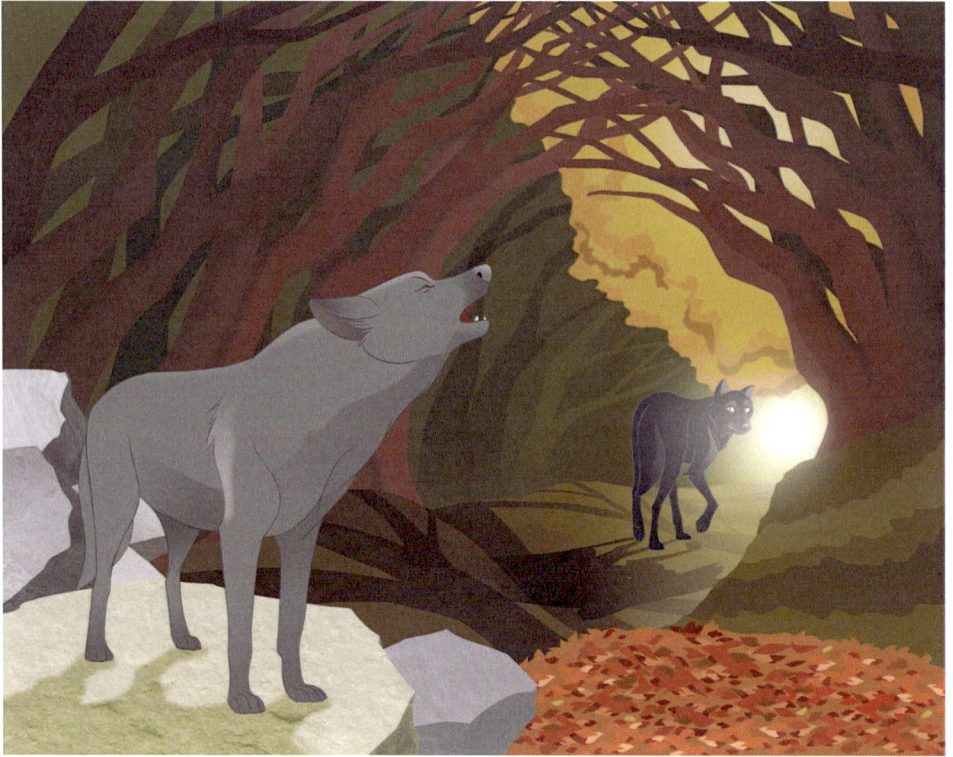

As the y<u>e</u>ars passed and Wolf #9 grew **old**er, one of her **daugh**ters took <u>o</u>ver the pack. It did not **ap**p<u>e</u>ar that things were **ver**y good **be**tw<u>ee</u>n the **moth**er and **daugh**ter. S<u>o</u>, Wolf #9 **end**ed up **leav**ing to **ven**ture **in**to the w<u>i</u>lds of **Wy**<u>o</u>**ming**. There, sh<u>e</u> **be**came a **found**ing **mem**ber of the **Bea**<u>r</u>tooth pack, **l**<u>o</u>c<u>a</u>t**ed** in the **Sh**<u>o</u>sh<u>o</u>**ne** **For**est. To this d<u>a</u>y, the **Bea**<u>r</u>tooth pack is **go**<u>o</u>ing strong!

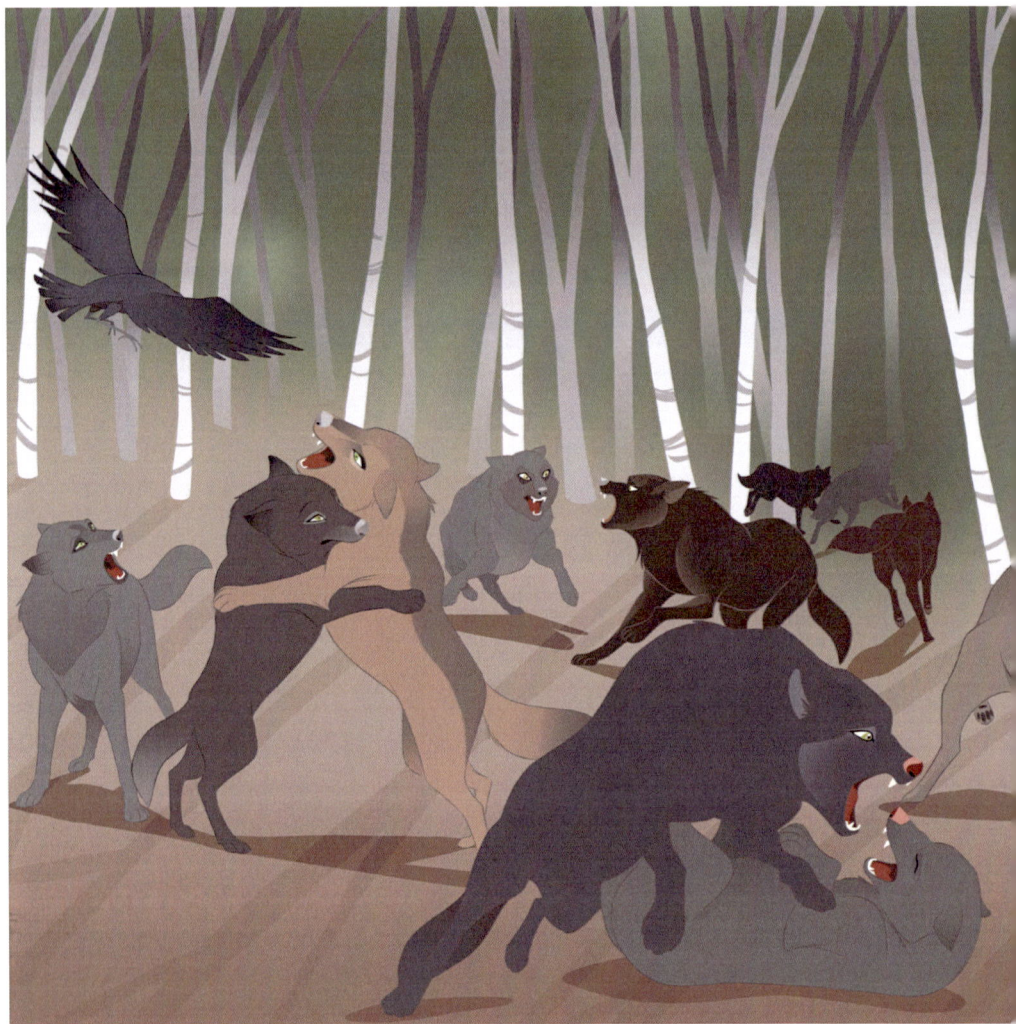

Since n**o** **o**rig**i**nal **mem**bers of the R**o**se Cr**ee**k Pack **re**ma**i**ned, the Wolf **Proj**ect **re**na**m**ed the pack, R**o**se Cr**ee**k 2. This pack **exp**e**ri**enced **con**flicts with the **Dr**u**i**d P**ee**ak Pack, which is the **larg**est pack in the park's **his**tory. The R**o**se Cr**ee**k Pack **e**ven**tu**ally br**o**ke **a**part and **dis**solved.

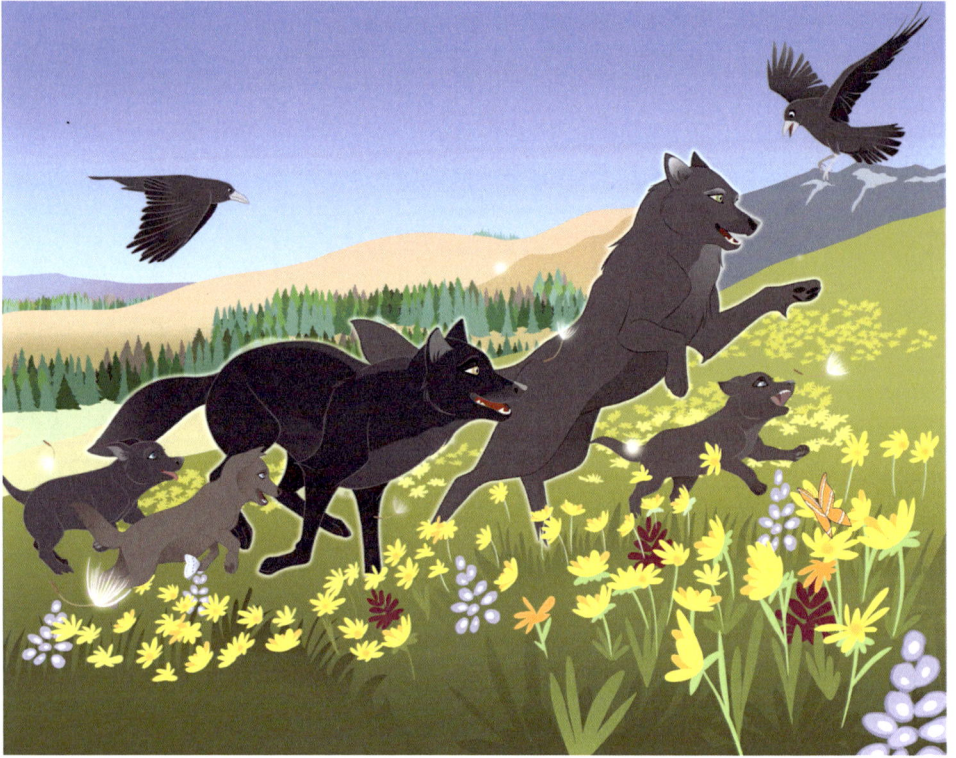

Wolf #9 and Wolf #7 f**a**ced **man**y **chal**leng**es**, from their **fam**ily b**e**ing torn **a**part in **Can**ada to the **strug**gle of **start**ing a new l**i**fe in **Yel**l**o**w**stone**. **To**geth**er**, they **be**c**a**me the **foun**d**a**t**ion** of the **lead**ing **ge**net**ic** l**i**ne in **Yel**l**o**w**stone**, with Wolf #9 con**t**rib**u**ting a **sig**nific**an**t **per**cent**age** of the g**e**nes.

What **mag**nif**i**cent wolves,
The **Ma**tri**archs** of
Yell**o**w**stone** **Na**tion**al** Park!

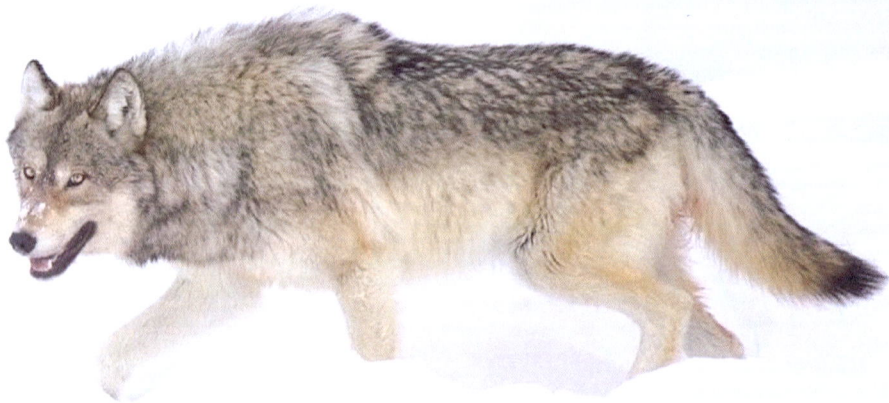
©Tin Man Lee

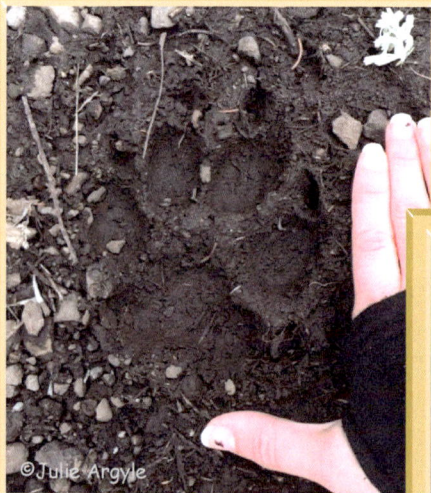
©Julie Argyle

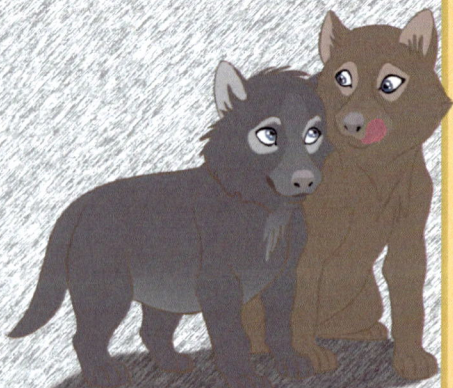
©Julie Argyle

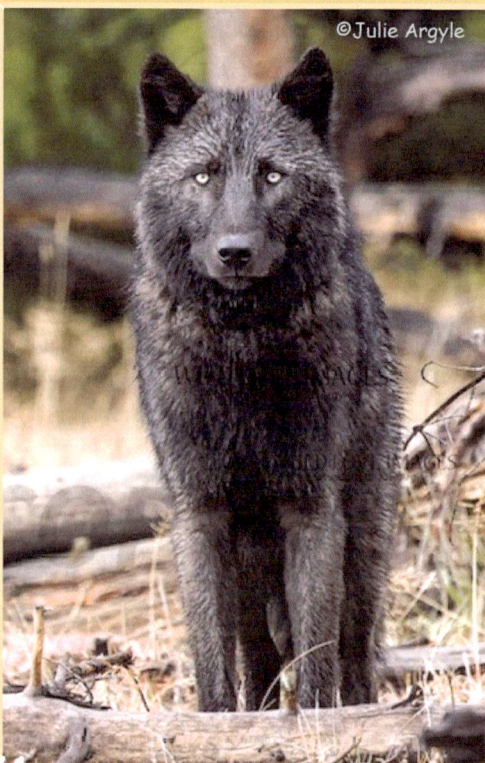

Gray Wolves

The gray wolf's **scientif**ic name is **Can**is **lu**pus.

In the **Un**ited States, there are **sev**eral types of wolf **spe**cies. The **Mexican** Wolf is a sub-**spe**cies of the Gray Wolf, while the Red Wolf is a **different spe**cies **al**together.

Yellow**stone** is home to the Gray Wolf!

- Wolves have scent glands on their tails and **be**tween their toes, **allowing** them to leave their scent **eve**ry time they walk! The scent they leave **be**hind **all**ows their **family** or friends to find them! They **also** leave their scent through their poop and pee!

- Wolves have **fan**tas**tic hear**ing and can hear four times **bet**ter than **hu**mans. So, if you hike in **Yel**low**stone**, you may not see **an**y wolves **be**cause they can hear you **com**ing, and they like to **a**void **peo**ple.

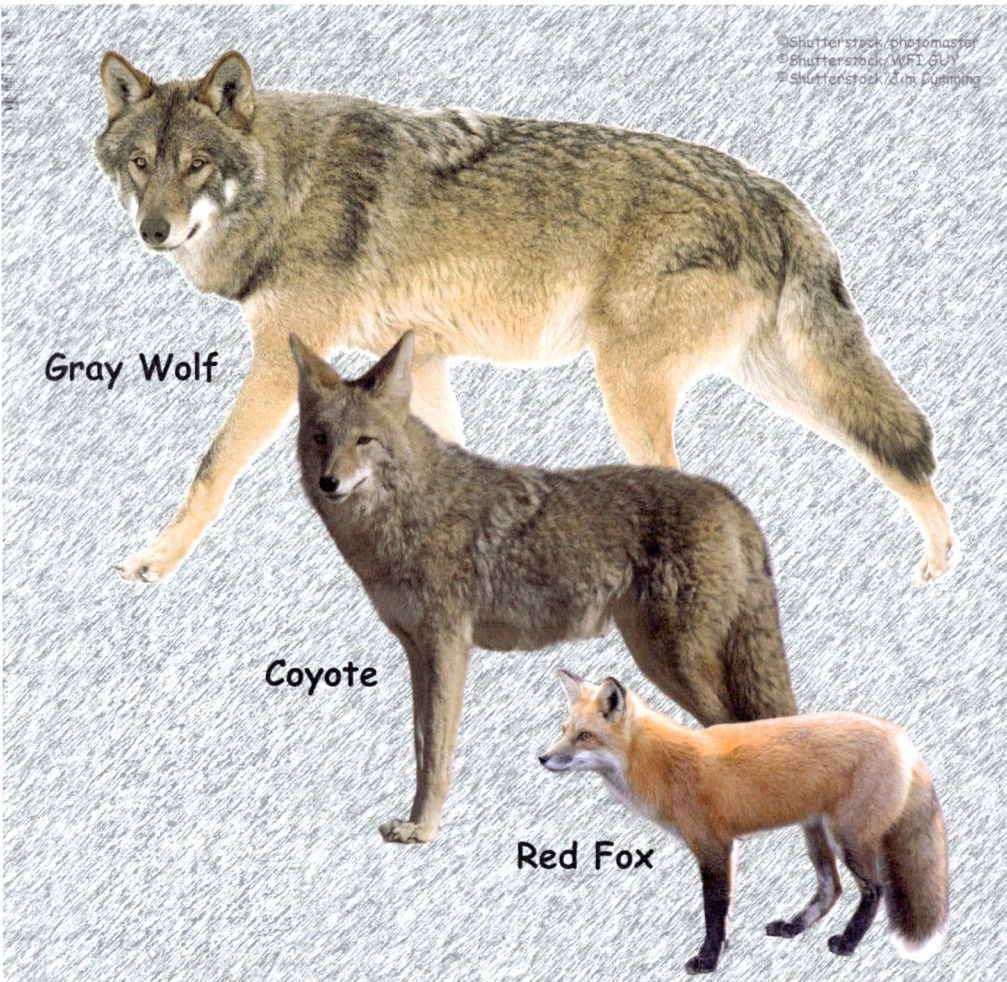

Gray Wolf

Coyote

Red Fox

	Length (Nose to Tail Tip)	Ear Shape	Snout Shape	Fur Color	Paw Size
Gray Wolf	5 to 6.5 ft.	small to medium, triangular, cupped	broad	gray, white, black, and/or brown	4 x 5 in.
Coyote	3.3 to 4.3 ft.	tall pointed	narrow	gray, brown, or red	2 x 2.5 in.
Red Fox	1 to 1.5 ft.	tall pointed	pointed	red with white tip on tails	2 x 1.5 in.

Gray Wolf **A**nat**o**my

The Gr<u>a</u>y Wolves of **Yell<u>o</u>wst<u>o</u>ne** are Big!

- **Fe**m<u>a</u>le wolves weigh 70 to 140 pounds, wh<u>i</u>le m<u>a</u>les can weigh 100 to 150 pounds. That's as big as an **av**er**age** man's weight!
- Gr<u>a</u>y wolves have **bea<u>u</u>ti**ful**, thick c<u>o</u>ats that k<u>ee</u>p them warm in the **win**ter.
- In **Yell<u>o</u>wst<u>o</u>ne**, the wolf's c<u>o</u>ats are **m<u>ai</u>n**ly black or gr<u>a</u>y.

If yo<u>u</u> g<u>o</u> **search**ing for wolves in the park, you may be **fort**u**nate** enough to **ex**p<u>e</u>r<u>i</u>ence a "thr<u>ee</u>-dog d<u>a</u>y!"

What does that m<u>ea</u>n?
Are there thr<u>ee</u> dogs **run**ning
around in **Yell<u>o</u>wst<u>o</u>ne**?

N<u>o</u>pe – not thr<u>ee</u> dogs – three dog types:
A Gr<u>a</u>y Wolf, a **Coy<u>o</u>te</u>**, and a Fox!

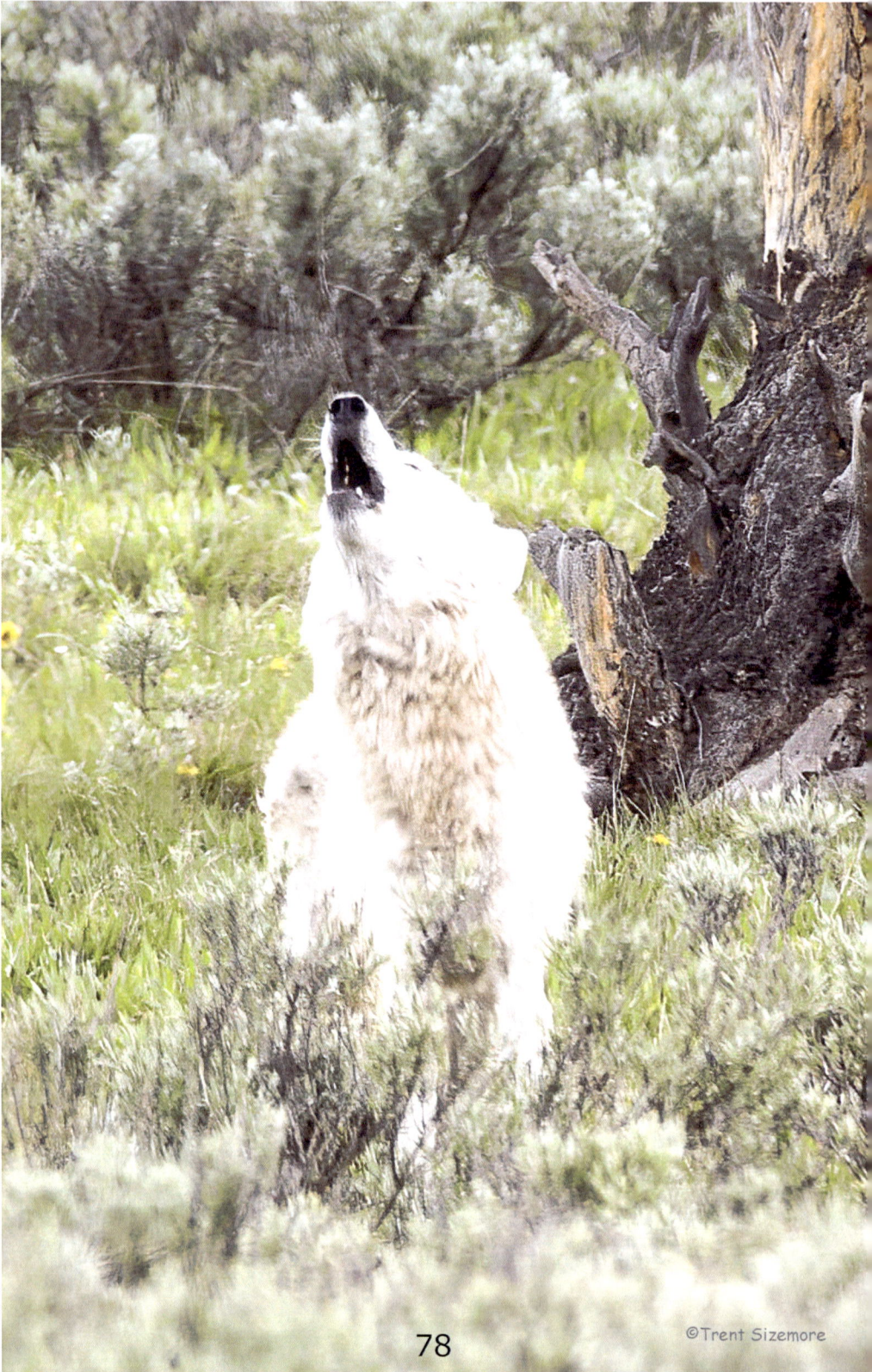

©Trent Sizemore

Did You Know That Wolves Talk to Each **Oth**er by **Howl**ing?

Yo**u** pick up the ph<u>o</u>ne, when yo<u>u</u> talk to **some**one, r<u>i</u>ght? Not wolves – they d<u>o</u>n't have ph<u>o</u>nes!

They howl!

They can talk to more than one wolf at a t<u>i</u>me since they can do a gro<u>u</u>p howl! **Different sp<u>e</u>**ci<u>e</u>s of wolves have **v<u>a</u>rious** types of howls that they <u>u</u>se for **different purp**os**es**. They can howl loud and long s<u>o</u> that **oth**ers can h<u>e</u>ar them from far **a**w<u>a</u>y.

Wolves howl:
- To find <u>e</u>ach **oth**er,
- To warn a **wan**der**ing** wolf that it m<u>a</u>y b<u>e</u> **en**ter**ing** their **ter**ritor**y**,
- To s<u>o</u>cial<u>i</u>**ze** with one **an**oth**er**,
- To pl<u>a</u>y tricks on **oth**er wolf packs. For **ex**am**ple**, a **small**er pack m<u>a</u>y howl **ver**y loud, **m<u>a</u>k**ing a r<u>i</u>val pack **be**li<u>e</u>ve that their pack **num**bers are **larg**er than they **re**ally are.

79

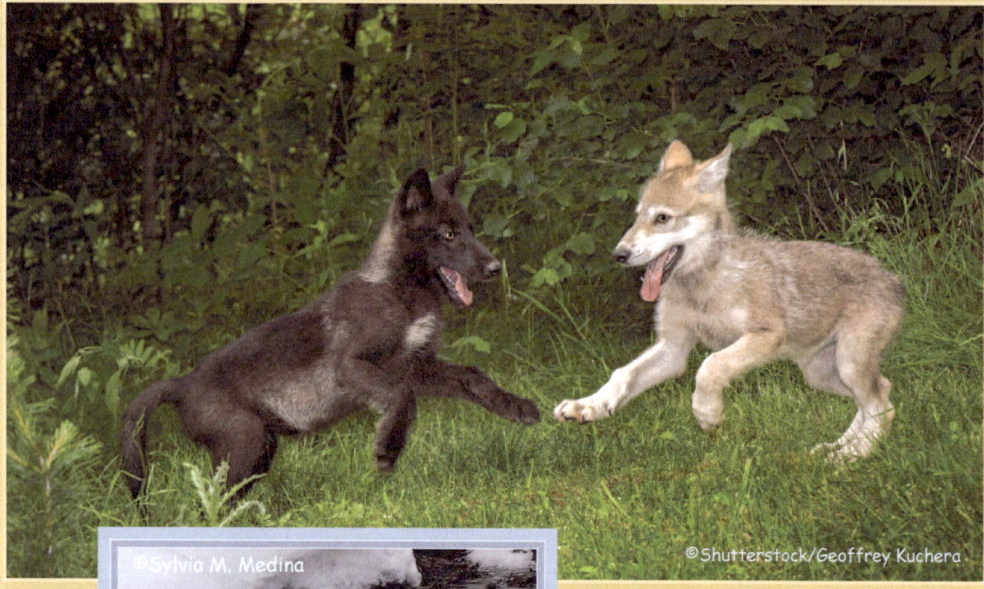
©Shutterstock/Geoffrey Kuchera

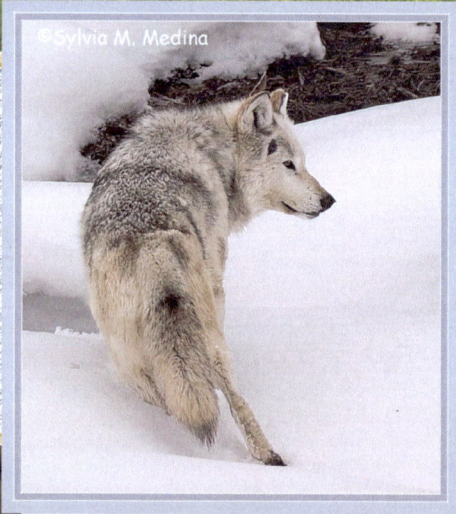
©Sylvia M. Medina

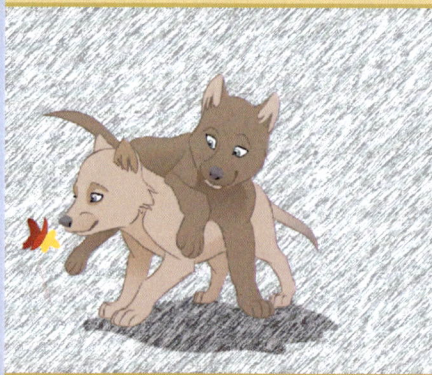

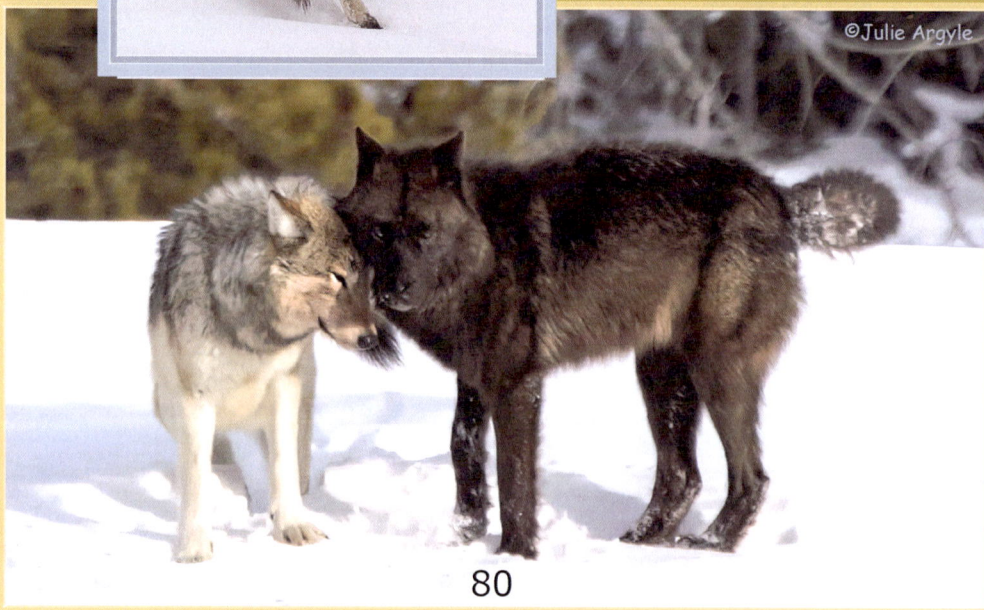
©Julie Argyle

80

Wolf **Attrib**__utes__ and **Be**havior

- All dogs come from **pre**historic wolves.
- Wolves **of**ten act like your dog!
- They play **to**gether, **cha**sing, and **romp**ing with each **oth**er.
- They show love and **af**fec**tion** by **lick**ing and **nuz**zling each **oth**er.

But just **be**cause wolves **re**sem**ble** dogs, does that mean you can try to pet one?

No, keep your **dis**tance and give them their space, they are wild **animals**!

In **Yel**low**stone**, you must stay at least 25 yards away from them.

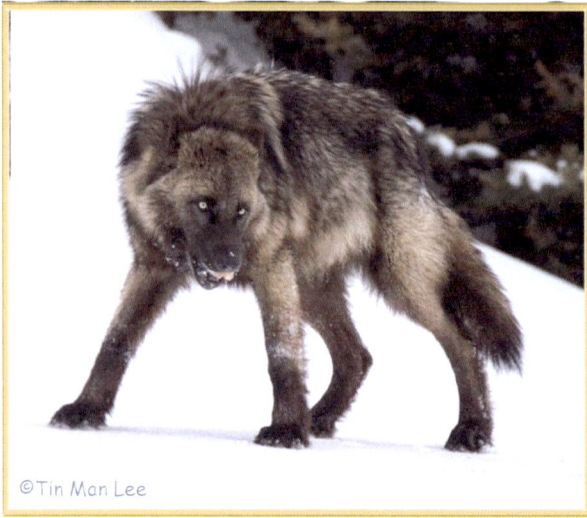
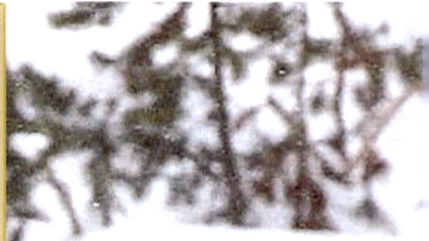

©Tin Man Lee

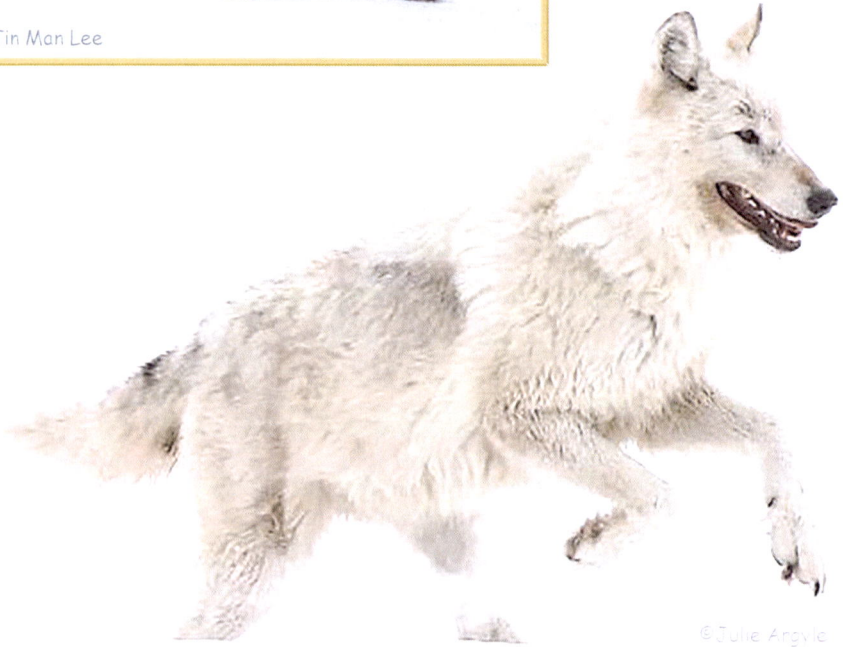

©Julie Argyle

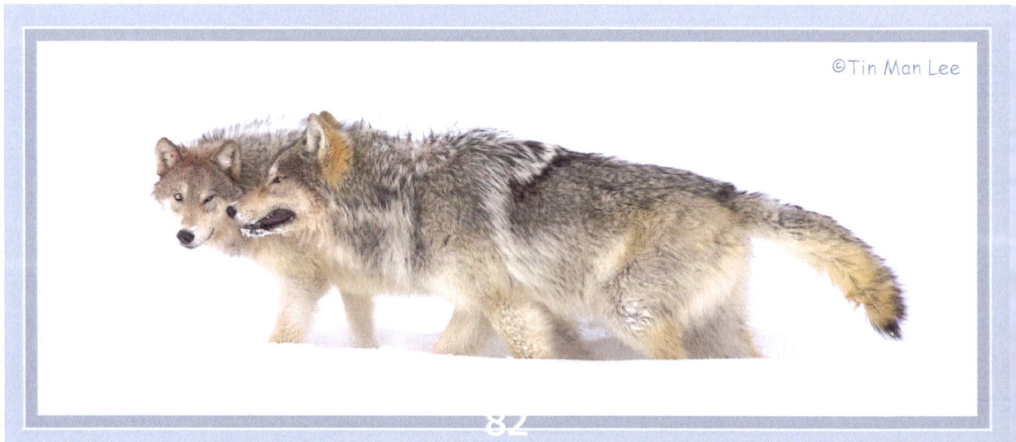

©Tin Man Lee

Wolves <u>E</u>ven Flirt with <u>E</u>ach **Oth**er

Fem<u>a</u>le wolves will prance **a**round **try**ing to **at**tract a m<u>a</u>le wolf. Wh<u>i</u>le a m<u>a</u>le wolf will run up and try to get her **at**ten**tion**!

When wolves are **be**ing **ag**gres**sive** or **sho**wing **dominance**, they will lift their t<u>a</u>il.

When they are **be**ing **sub**mis**sive** to **an**oth**er** wolf, they crouch or **lo**wer their t<u>a</u>il!

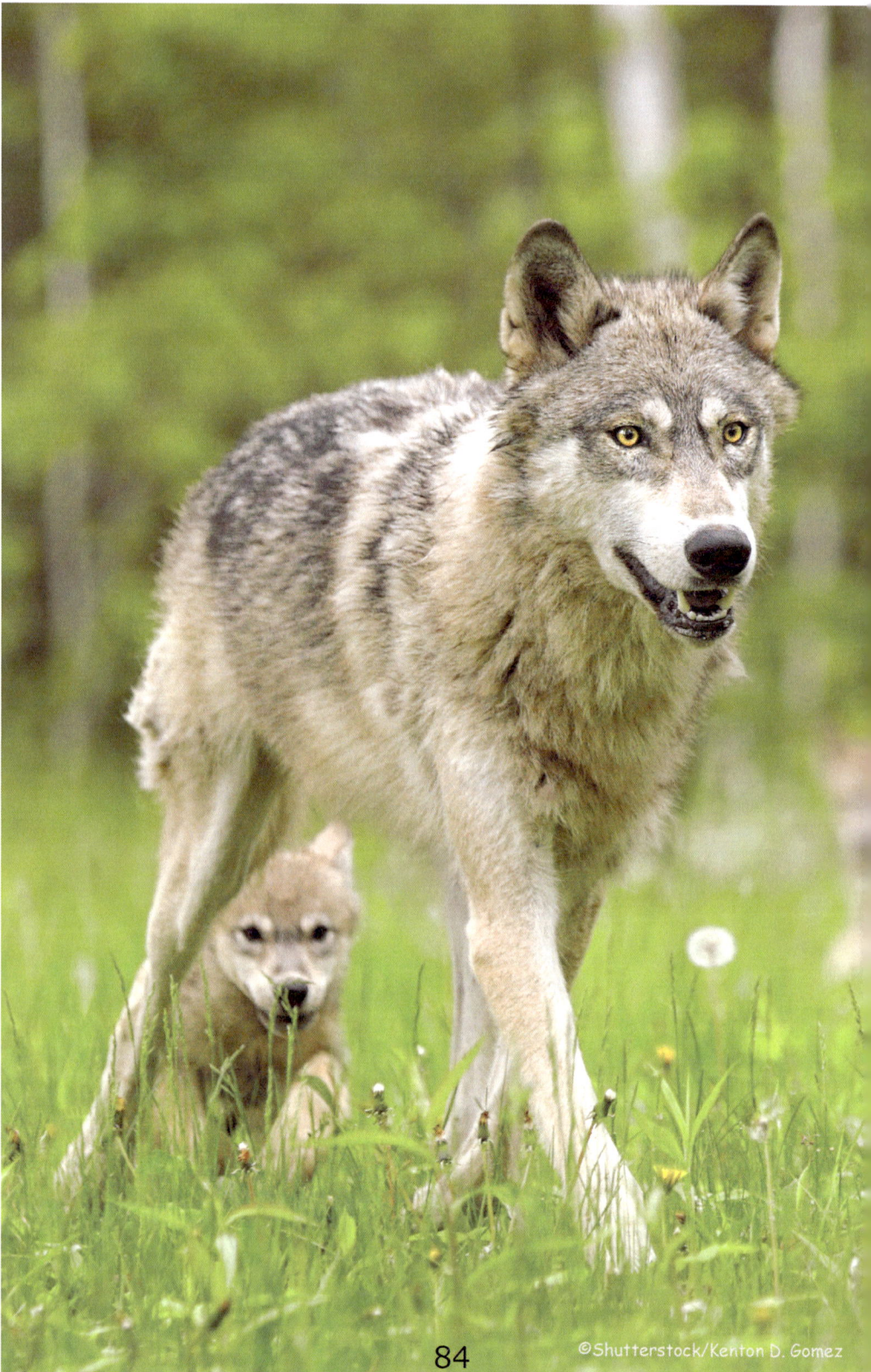

©Shutterstock/Kenton D. Gomez

Wolf **Families**!

Wolf **families** are called packs!

They are a lot like ours!

- The wolf **family** includes a **moth**er (**al**pha female), a **fa**ther (**al**pha male), and **broth**ers and **sis**ters.
- **Some**times, they may have **an**other friend or **cou**sin as part of the **family**.
- A friend or **family mem**ber will **of**ten help **ba**by**sit** the pups when mom and dad go away to hunt; they are called **nan**ny wolves!
- **Moth**er wolves can have up to six pups, which are usually born around April. The **ba**by wolves drink their **moth**er's milk **un-** til they are about five weeks old when they start the **wean**ing **pro**cess (the **maximum** litter size is eleven pups).
- Wolf pups are **al**so born with **beau**tiful blue colored eyes, but their eye **col**or **chang**es as they grow older!

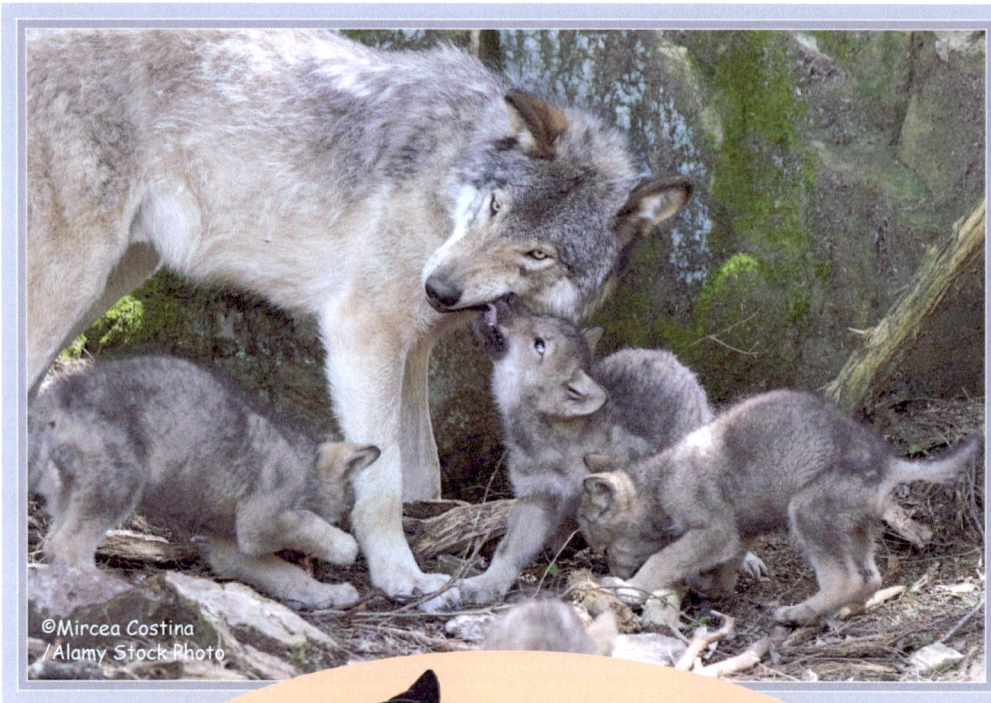
©Mircea Costina
/Alamy Stock Photo

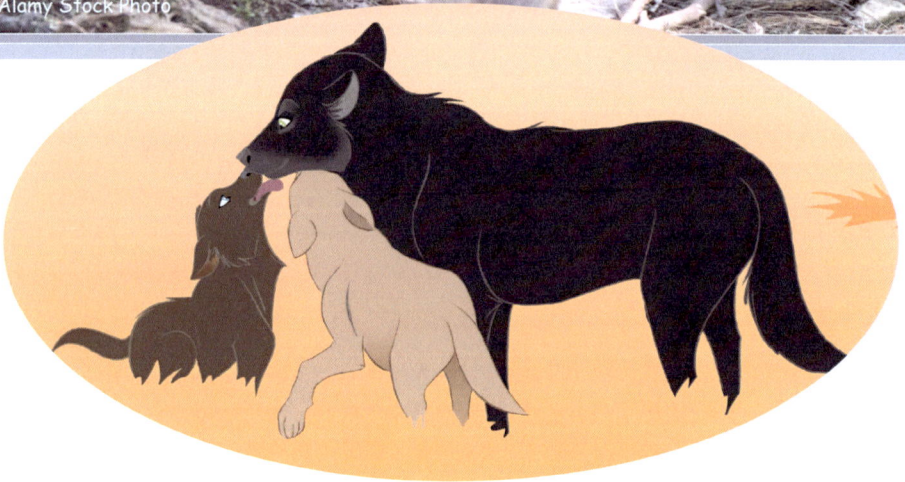

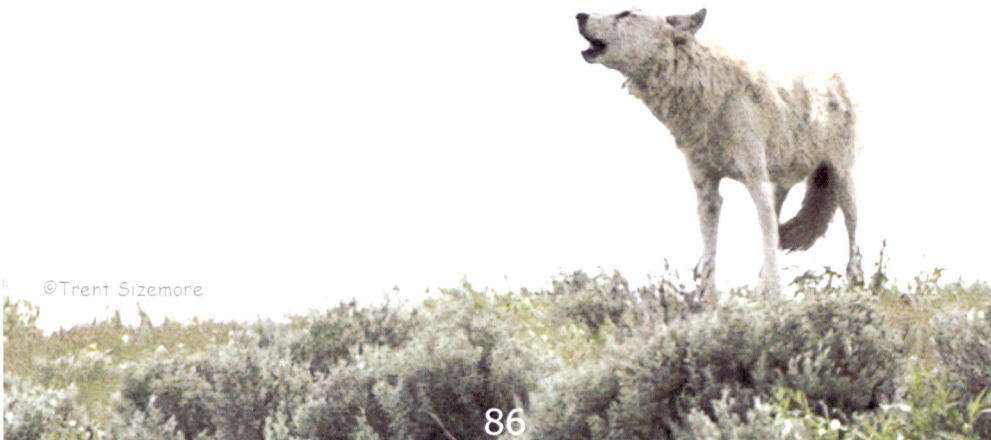
©Trent Sizemore

86

- When wolves f<u>ee</u>d their pups, they will g<u>o</u> out to hunt for a m<u>ea</u>l. **Up**on **re**turn**ing**, they **re**gurg**i**t<u>a</u>te the m<u>ea</u>t, **m<u>ea</u>n**ing they will thr<u>o</u>w it back up, and the pups will <u>ea</u>t it.
- Yo<u>u</u> m<u>i</u>ght think this is **yuck**y – but not the pups – they love it!

> Did yo<u>u</u> kn<u>o</u>w that dogs have
> **mem**or<u>ie</u>s of b<u>e</u>ing fed as pups?
> When they lick your f<u>a</u>ce, they m<u>a</u>y b<u>e</u> **try**ing
> to get yo<u>u</u> to **re**gurg**i**t<u>a</u>te food for them!

When an **al**pha **moth**er wolf d<u>i</u>es, the pack **of**ten **strug**gles to st<u>a</u>y **to**geth**er** b<u>e</u>cause sh<u>e</u> is the pack **l<u>ea</u>d**er. While **an**y **l<u>ea</u>d**ers death can have an **im**pact, the loss of the **al**pha **fe**m<u>a</u>le is worst.

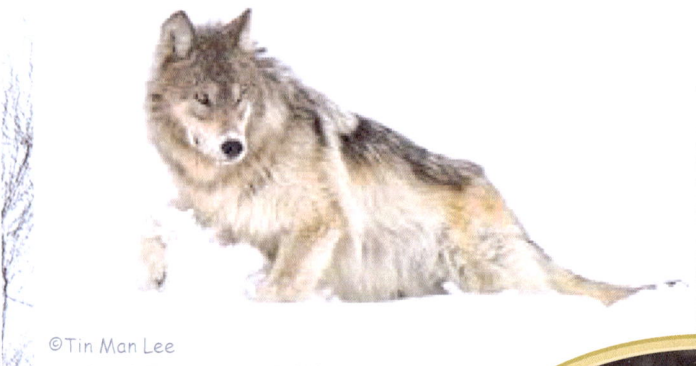
©Tin Man Lee

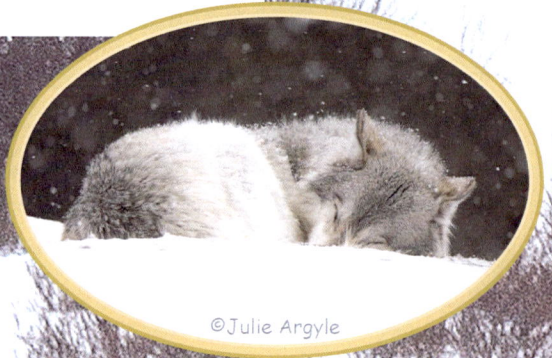
©Julie Argyle

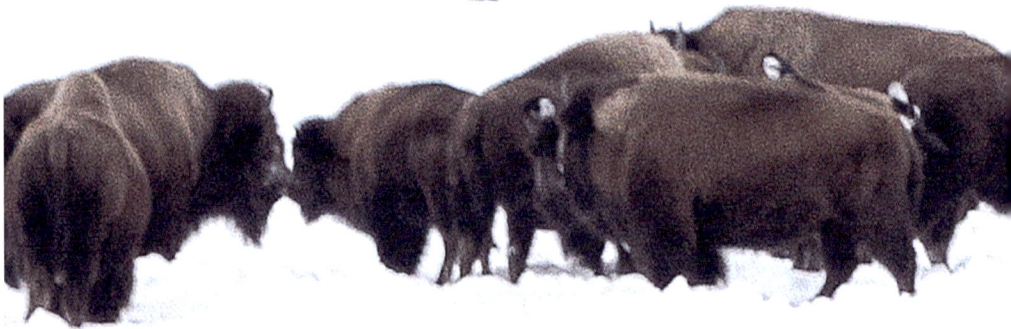

©Trent Sizemore

How Do Wolves Survive?

Yellowstone wolves have quite the life!
They LOVE the cold!

The **environ**ment in the park is **ex**treme
and can range from **ver**y cold **frig**id
temperatures **rang**ing from 40 **de**grees
below **Fah**ren**heit** in **win**ter to **ver**y hot in the
summer. They have thick, warm coats with
two **lay**ers and their feet do not get cold.

What do they eat?

To feed **them**selves, wolves must hunt!
They **of**ten hunt in packs when **target**ing
large **animals** like **bi**son or elk. They **al**so feed
on **small**er **animals** such as ground **squir**rels,
marmots, **rab**bits, voles, and even **bea**vers.

Wolves have **su**per night **vi**sion, which
helps them have **suc**cess**ful** hunts **dur**ing the
darker hours, dusk and **sun**rise.

They can **trav**el up to 30 miles per day!

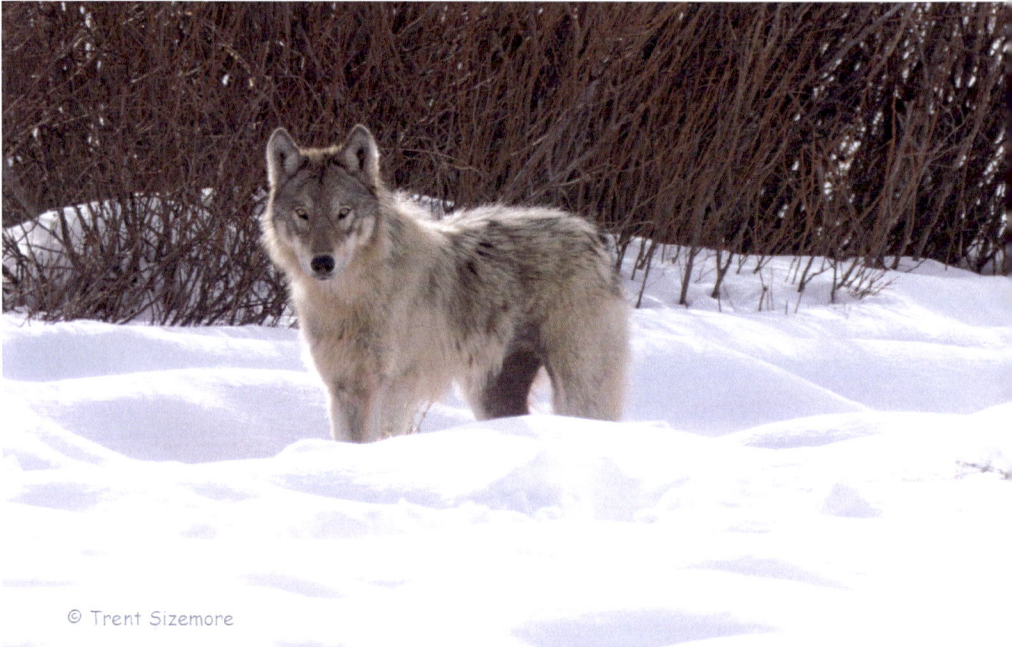

© Trent Sizemore

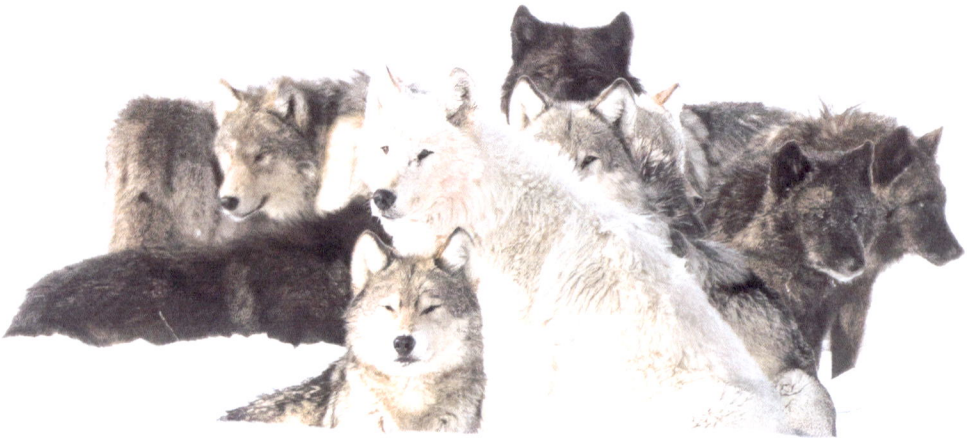

© Trent Sizemore

The Life Span of a Wolf
in **Yellowstone**

- When a wolf leaves its pack and **en**ters **an**oth**er** pack's **ter**ri**tor**y, the **resident** wolves will **fierce**ly **pro**tect their home and may run the lone wolf off or kill it. This is the **pri**m**ary** way wolves die in **Yellowstone**.

- Wolves **typ**ic**al**ly live for **a**bout 4 to 5 years.

- **How**ev**er**, some wolves have beat the odds. Wolf #907, the famed one-eyed **al**pha **fe**male of the **Junc**tion Butte Pack, **re**cent**ly** died while **de**fend**ing** her **fam**ily. At 11 years old, she was **re**cent**ly** the **old**est **liv**ing wolf in **Yellowstone**. **Throug**hout her life, she gave birth to nine **lit**ters of pups.

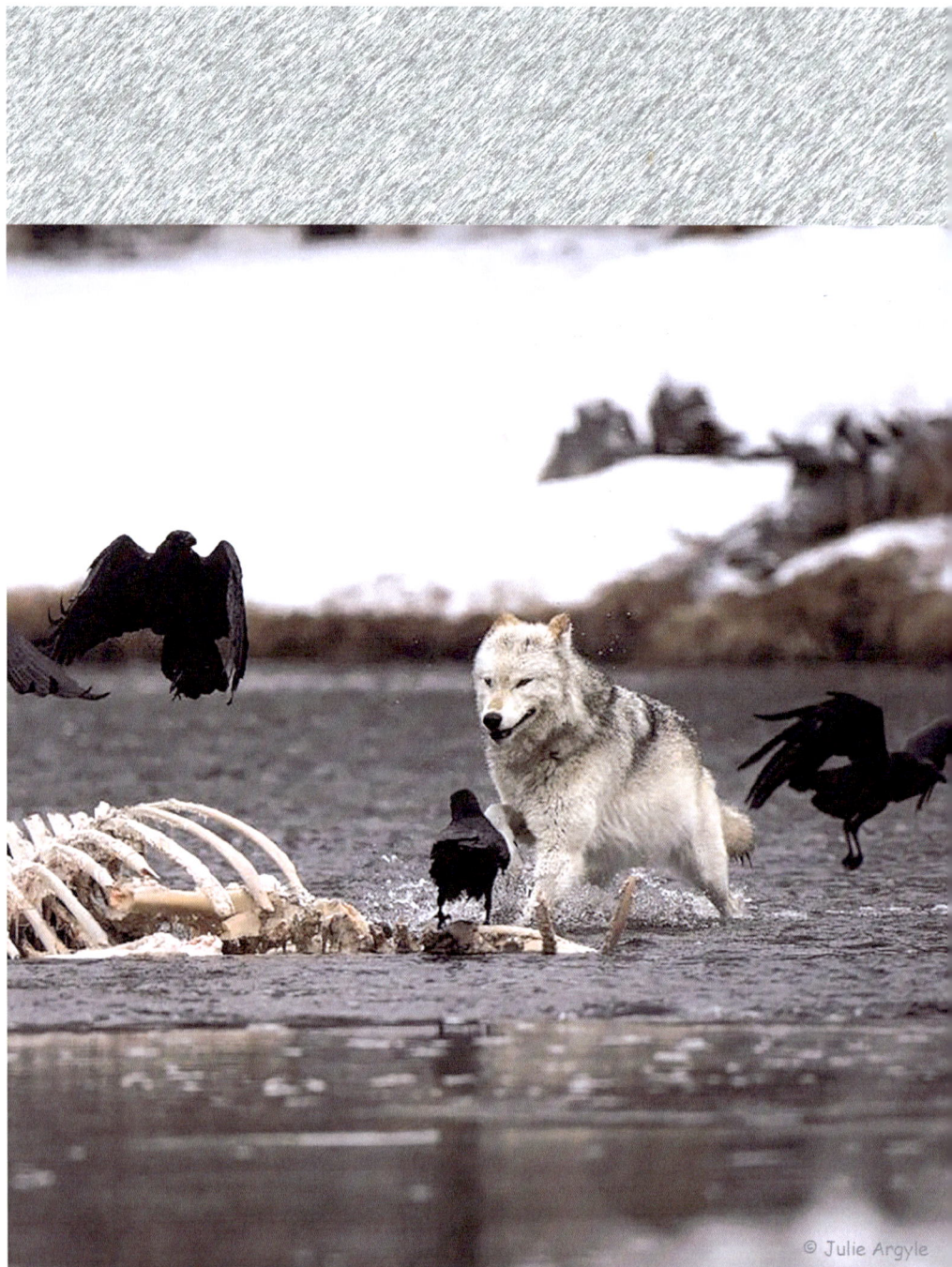

© Julie Argyle

Why Do Yo<u>u</u> S<u>ee</u> **Ra**vens **A**round Wolves?

Wolf hunts **gen**era**l**ly l<u>e</u>ave **left<u>o</u>vers** from their kill. S<u>o</u>, **ra**vens, tend to **fol**l<u>o</u>w the wolves, **h<u>o</u>p**ing they can get a snack **af**ter the wolves have **fin**ished **<u>ea</u>t**ing.

There is <u>e</u>ven a **doc<u>u</u>ment**ed c<u>a</u>se where **ra**vens have been s<u>ee</u>n **play**ing with wolf pups!

Ravens just want to have fun (and <u>ea</u>t)!

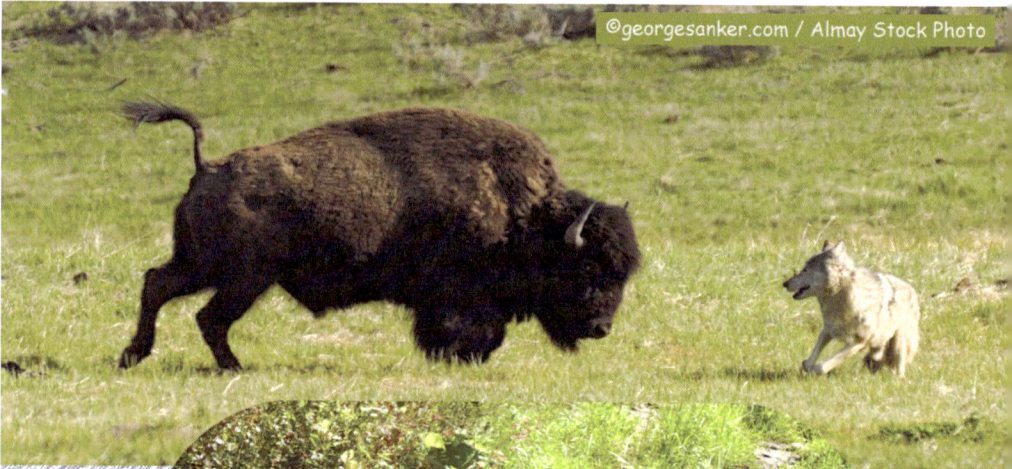

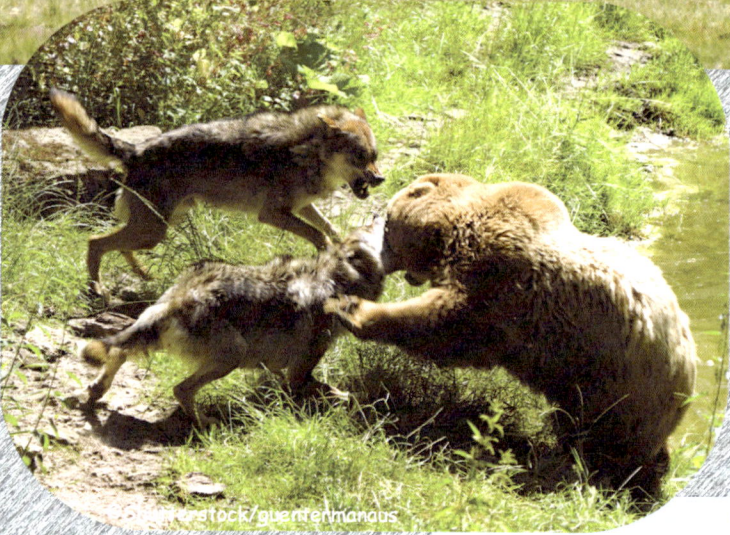

©georgesanker.com / Almay Stock Photo

©Shutterstock/guentermanaus

©Leo Leckie

©Trent Sizemore

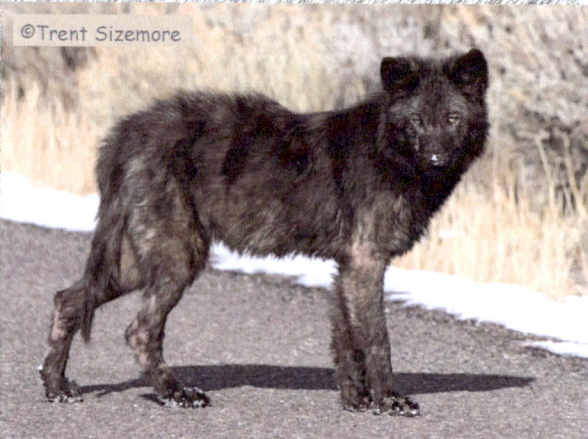

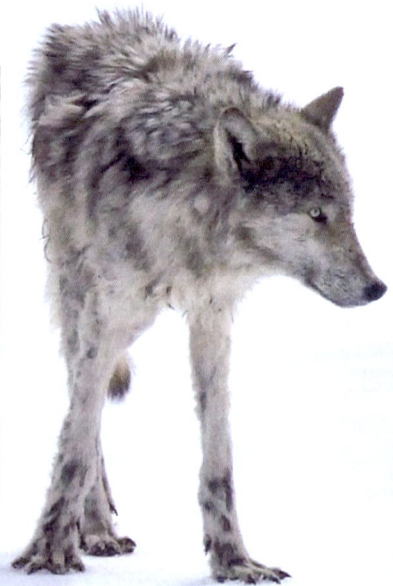

Do Wolves Have **Enemies**?

Yes, they do. Their main **enemies** are **hu**mans who hunt and poach them.

Other **enemies in**clude large **animals** like **bi**son or elk, which can gore or kick them, as well as **griz**zlies, which may **at**tack them.

Mange

Mange is **also** one of their worst **enemies**! Mange is a **con**di**tion** caused by mites that **bur**row **in**to the wolf's skin. This **dis**ease leads to **in**tense **itch**ing and hair loss, which can **dis**cour**age** them from **hunt**ing. If they don't hunt, they can't eat, which can **re**sult in their death. If they get mange in the **win**ter, the loss of their fur **re**duc**es** the warmth their coat **pro**vides, and they may freeze to death.

*But one of their **great**est **enemies** comes from **ri**val wolves in **oth**er packs.*

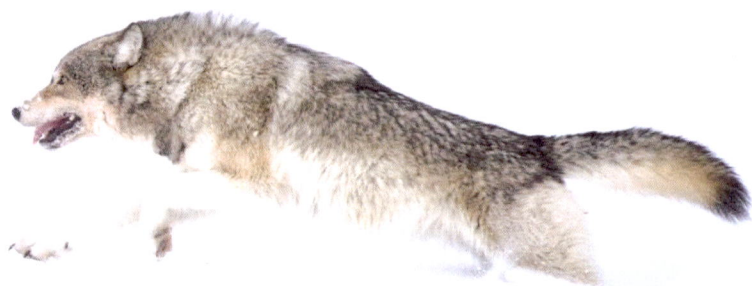

©Tin Man Lee

Current Wolf Protection and the Endangered Species Act

In the 19th and 20th **centuries**, the **government decided** to kill off all the wolves, and by 1950, **very** few **re**mained. In 1973, the **Endangered Species** Act was passed, **pro**tect**ing man**y types of **animals**, **inclu**d**ing** the wolves of **Yellowstone**.

The **re**intro**duction** of wolves to **Yellowstone** occurred in 1995. **However**, **af**ter **many** years, **changes** in the law **al**lowed **I**dah**o**, **Wyoming**, and **Mon**tana to hunt wolves.

Even th**ough** wolves **liv**ing in **Yellowstone** still have **protection**, once they **le**ave the park **boundaries**, **hunt**ers or **poach**ers can kill them.

If **Yellowstone** wolves could read the sign **say**ing, "**Yellowstone** Park **Boundary**," **I** doubt they would risk **cross**ing the park line.

97

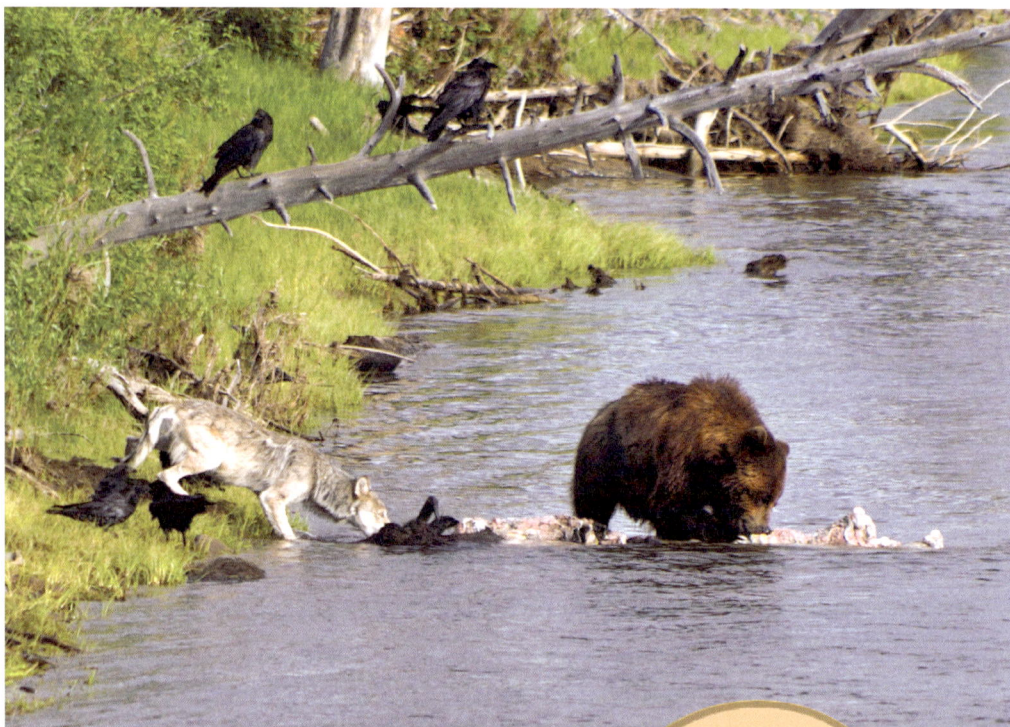

©Jonathan Eden / Alamy Stock Photo

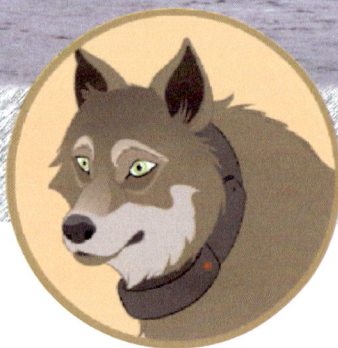

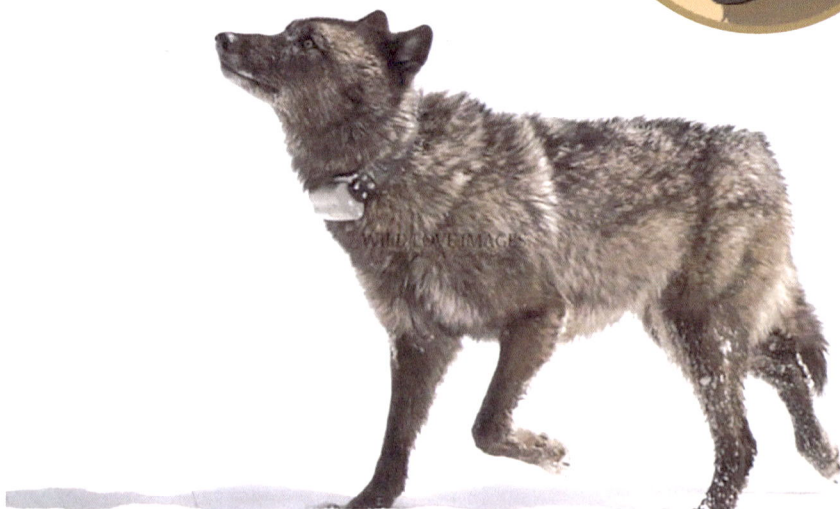

Reintroduction of Wolves to the Ecosystem

The **reintro**duction of wolves in **Yel**lowst**o**ne has led to the **form**a**tion** of new packs, **allowing visitors** to s**ee** wolves in the park **to**d**ay**. **Be**fore the wolves **re**turned, **North**ern **Yel**lowst**o**ne had as **many** as 20,000 elk. In their search for food, the elk **be**gan to **o**ver**browse**, which **dam**aged the plants and tr**ee**s, **mak**ing the land **un**health**y**. When the wolves **re**turned, be**a**rs and **coug**ars **also re**app**eared**, and they **start**ed **hunt**ing the elk. This helped **de**creas**e** the elk **pop**u**la**tion and **re**store the park's **habit**at to its **pre**vious **health**y st**a**te. As a **re**sult, **oth**er **spe**ci**es**, such as **bea**vers and **na**tive plants l**i**ke **wil**l**o**ws and **as**pens, have **also re-**turned.

Collars: The **Yel**lowst**o**ne Wolf **Proj**ect **u**ses **Ver**y-High-**Fre**quen**cy** (VHF) and **Glob**al-**Position-Sig**nal (**GPS**) **col**lars to **gath**er wolf **da**ta. Th**ese** **col**lars **al**low the **proj**ect t**ea**m to track wolves' **lo**c**a**tions, **i**den**ti**fy the **num**ber of wolves in the park and **stud**y their **be**h**a**v**iors**.

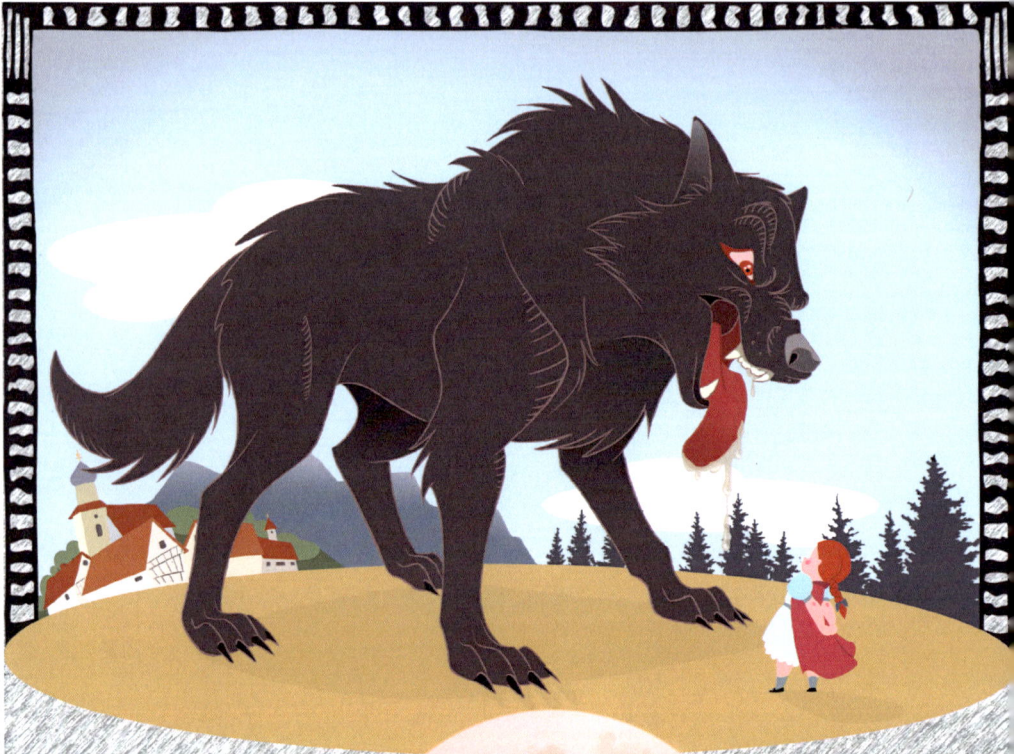

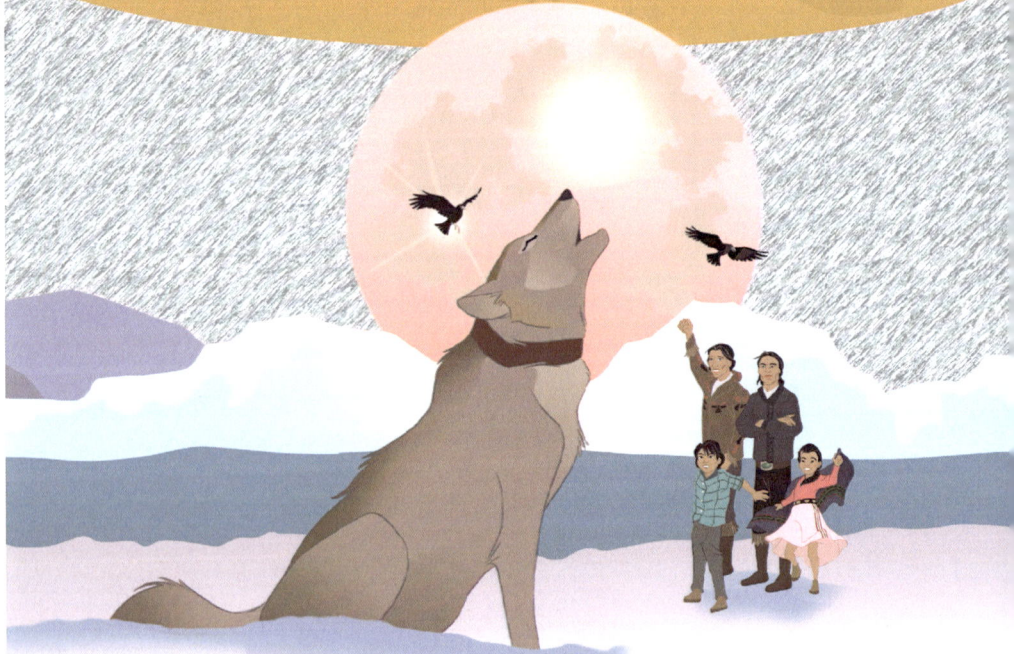

Why do Wolves Have a Bad Reputation?

In many Native cultures, the wolf is regarded as a spiritual guide and protector, symbolizing humility and courage. Often misunderstood, wolves are far from the evil creatures, as portrayed in stories like "Little Red Riding Hood."

In reality, they pose a minimal risk to humans and are not a significant competitor to hunters or major threats to cattle and sheep.

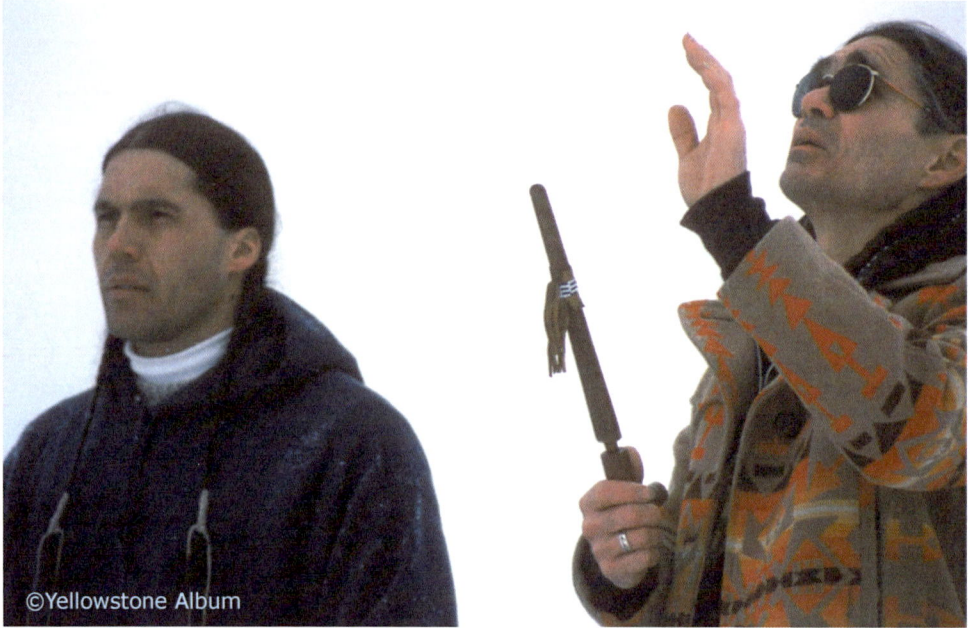

©Yellowstone Album

John **Pot**ter and Scott **Fra**zier

Native **A**meri**c**ans and their **Re**la**tion**ship with the Wolf

Our **Peo**ple fe**e**l a d**ee**p, **an**ces**tr**al t**i**e to Maa' **iin**gan (Wolf) as our First **Broth**er. Our **stor**i**e**s sp**e**ak of how **Cre**ator brought **O**rigi**n**al Man and Maa' **iin**gan **to**geth**er** when Man was **a**l**o**ne in the world and sought a **com**pan**ion**. **Cre**ator then g**a**ve them the task of **walk**ing the Earth **to**geth**er**, and of **giv**ing n**a**mes to all of His **Cre**a**tion**. In this w**a**y, they **be**came very close - **be**com**ing al**m**o**st as one. When Wolf and Man had **fin**ished with what **Cre**ator had asked, **Cre**ator t**o**ld them that they must now **sep**arate, and g**o** on to **be**gin their **o**wn **fam**ili**e**s and w**a**ys of l**i**fe - but to **re**mem**ber** and **hon**or that they would **AL**W**A**YS be **Broth**er to one **an**oth**er**. And m**o**st **im**por**tant**ly, **re**mem**ber** that what **hap**pens to one, will **al**s**o** **hap**pen to the **oth**er.

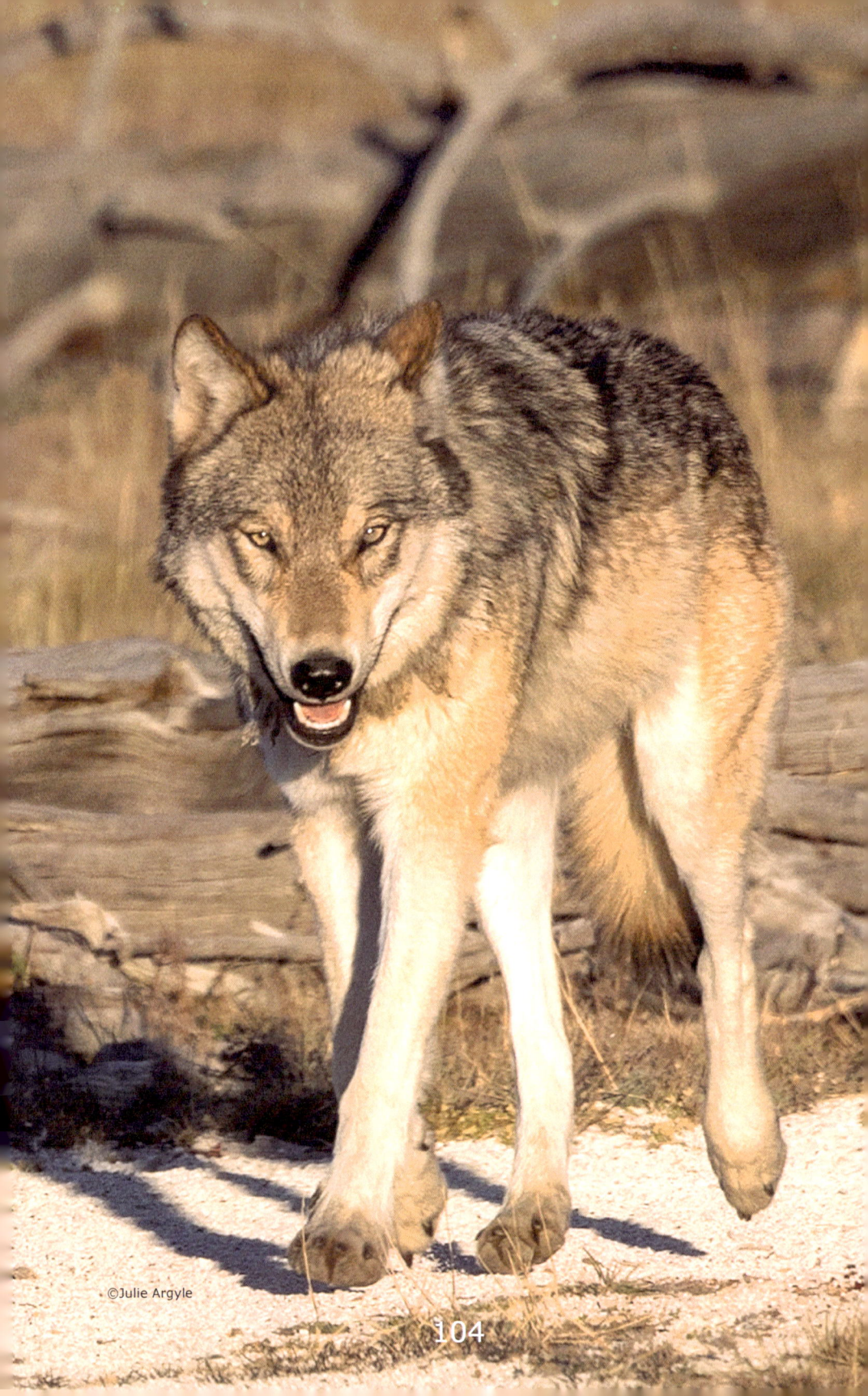

©Julie Argyle

So, in 1995 and 1996, my **broth**er Scott and I were asked by **Yellowstone National** Park to **per**form the **Cerem**ony for the **arrival** of Wolves **be**ing brought in from **Can**ada to **re**populate the Park with its most **important missing pres**ence. Of course we said "yes," **es**pe**cial**ly **be**cause some of these Wolves were **tak**en from their **families** and brought **hun**dreds of miles to a strange land. Since there's no such thing as "**or**phans" **a**mong **In**dians, we **per**formed **wel**com**ing** and **a**dop**tion Cerem**on**ies** for them - **teach**ing them our songs - since, in the **be**gin**ning**, it was Wolf who taught us, as **hu**mans, to find our own voice.

To this day, we go back **in**to the Park **eve**ry year to **hon**or our **ex**tend**ed family** of Wolves with song - for their **voic**es have **giv**en us life from the **be**gin**ning**.

John **Pot**ter's **peo**ple are the **O**jib**we** of **Up**per Great Lakes **Coun**try, **Wis**con**sin**. Scott **Fra**zier's **peo**ple are the Sioux/Crow.

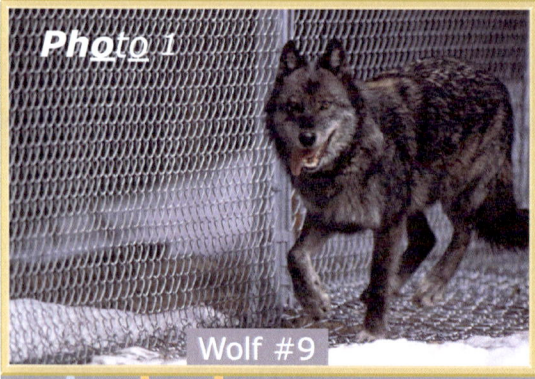
Photo 1
Wolf #9

The Rose Creek Pack
Photo **Al**bum

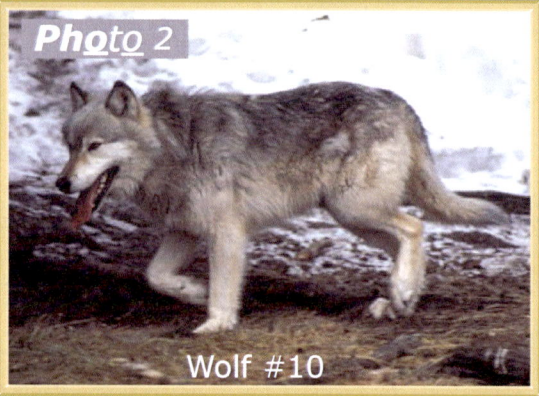
Photo 2
Wolf #10

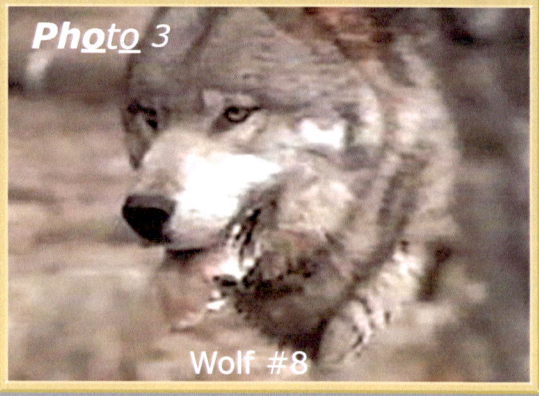
Photo 3
Wolf #8

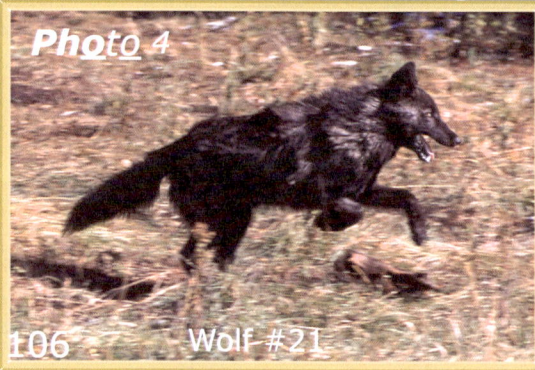
Photo 4
106   Wolf #21

To Wolf #7
Contin**u**ed on
Page 108

The **Re**al Wolves in this **Stor**y

*The R*o*se Cr*ee*k Pack*

***Ph**o*to** 1:* Wolf #9 **found**ed the R*o*se Cr*ee*k Pack. She was a **fe**m*a*le **al**pha who c*a*me from **Can**ada.

***Ph**o*to** 2:* Wolf #10 was the m*a*le **al**pha m*a*te of Wolf #9. He c*a*me from **Can**ada. Wolf #10 was the **fa**ther of Wolf #21.

***Ph**o*to** 3:* Wolf #8
After Wolf #10 was killed, Wolf #9 met Wolf #8, and he **a**dopt**ed** her pups. H*e* **al**s*o* r*a*ised Wolf #21 and taught him the **lead**er**ship** h*e* l*a*ter **dis**pl*a*yed.

***Ph**o*to** 4:* Wolf #21's **roy**alty c*a*me from Wolf #9 and #10's **un**ion. Wolf #21 was born and **be**c*a*me King of **La**mar **Val**l*e*y. H*e* was **fa**thered and **a**dopt**ed** by Wolf #8 **af**ter Wolf #10's death.

From Wolf #9
Continued
from Page 106

The **Leopold** Pack
Photo **Al**bum

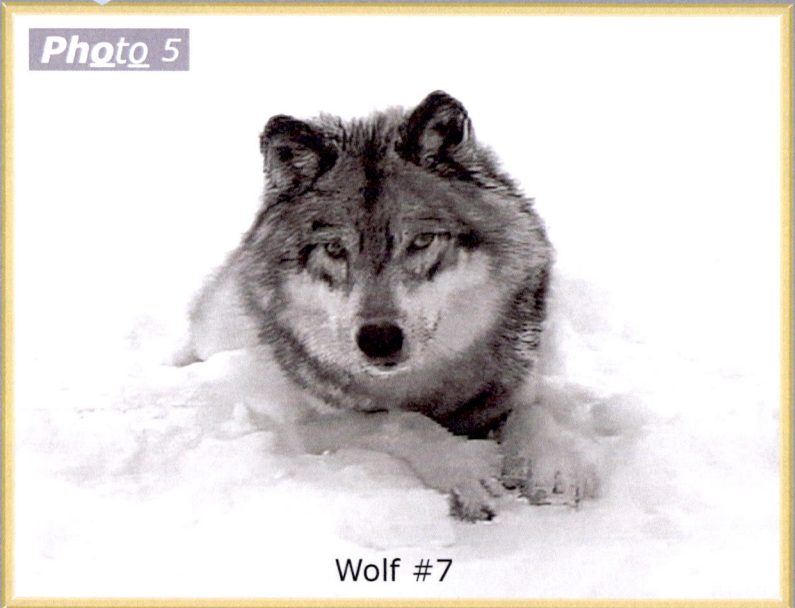

*Pho*to 5

Wolf #7

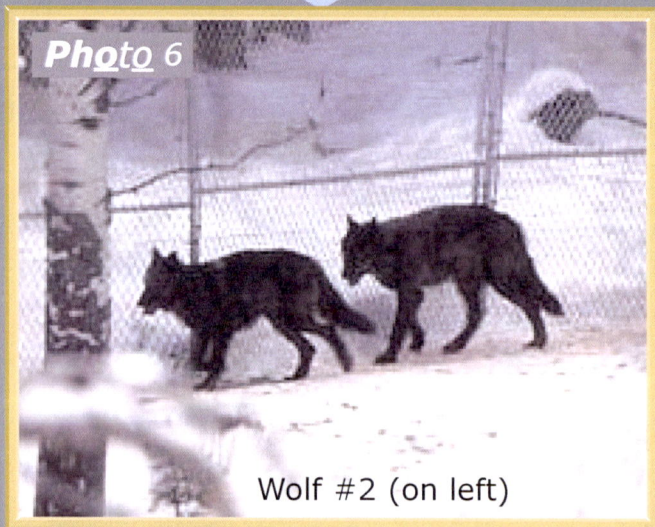

*Pho*to 6

Wolf #2 (on left)

The **Re**al Wolves in this **Stor**y
*The **Le**o**pold** Pack!*

***Pho**to 5:* Wolf #7 was a **daugh**ter of Wolf #9. Wolf #7 **found**ed and was the **al**pha **fe**male of the **Le**o**pold** pack. The **Le**o**pold** pack was **lo**cat**ed** n**ea**r **Ge**ode Cr**ee**k.

***Pho**to 6:* Wolf #2 and Wolf #7 r**ai**sed up to 25 pups to at l**ea**st one y**ea**r of **a**ge! They st**a**yed **to**geth**er** for **o**ver **sev**en y**ea**rs and **re**m**ai**ned **fa**ith**ful** to **ea**ch **oth**er!

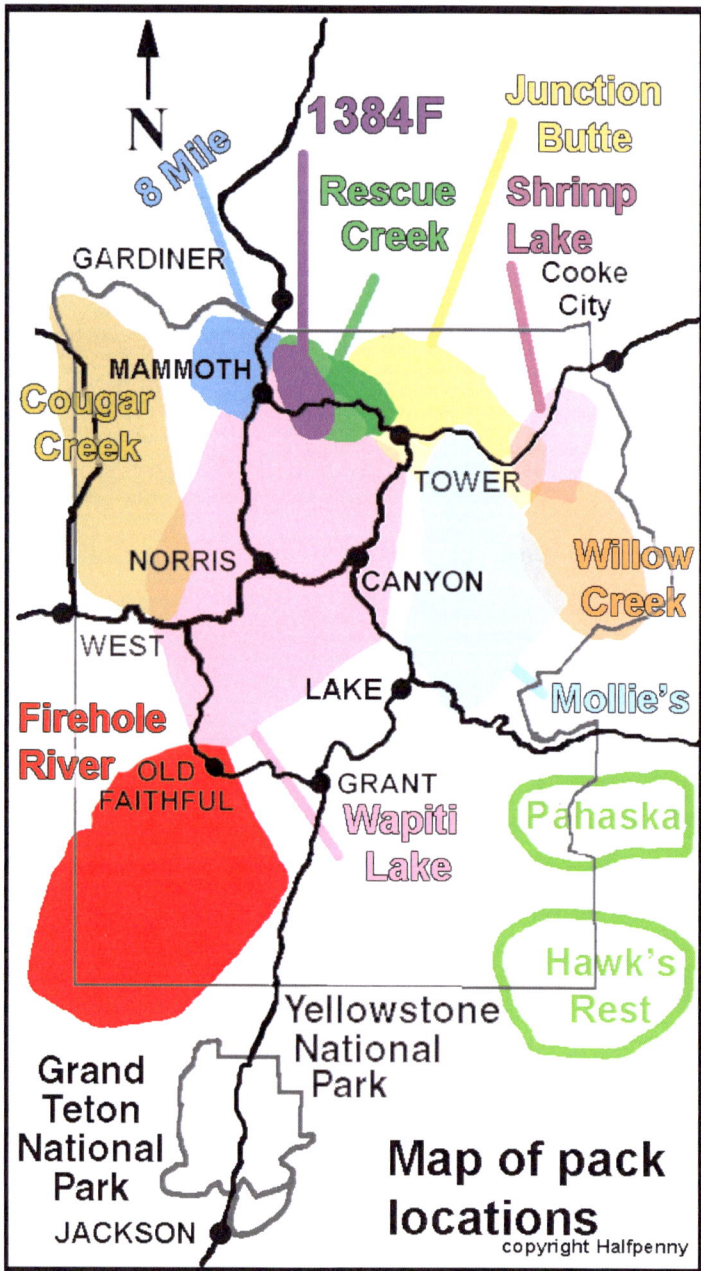

Map of pack locations

copyright Halfpenny

Pahaska and Hawks Rest packs are officially Wyoming packs but they roam into Yellowstone National Park occasionally.

Wolf Pack map provided by Jim Halfpenny.

110

Yel**lowstone** Wolves

Estab**lish** Their **Terri**tori**es**

As of **Jan**u**a**ry 2024, there were **ap**prox**i**matel**y** 124 wolves **liv**ing in Yel**lowstone Na**tion**al** Park.

They live in 10 packs:

- **Wap**iti L**a**ke
- **Junc**tion B**u**tte
- **Mol**lie's
- **Res**c**u**e Cr**ee**k
- **Cou**gar Cr**ee**k
- Shrimp L**a**ke
- **Wil**l**ow** Cr**ee**k
- **Fi**re**ho**le **Riv**er
- 1384F Gro**u**p
- 8 M**i**le

Trans-**Bound**ary Packs

- **Pa**has**ka**
- Hawk's Rest

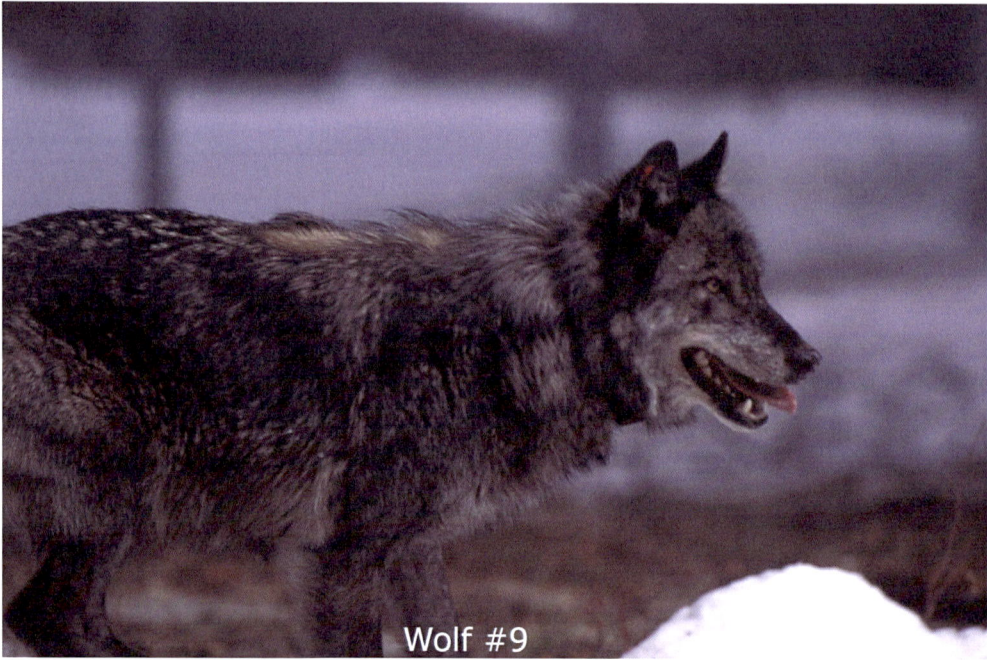

Wolf #9

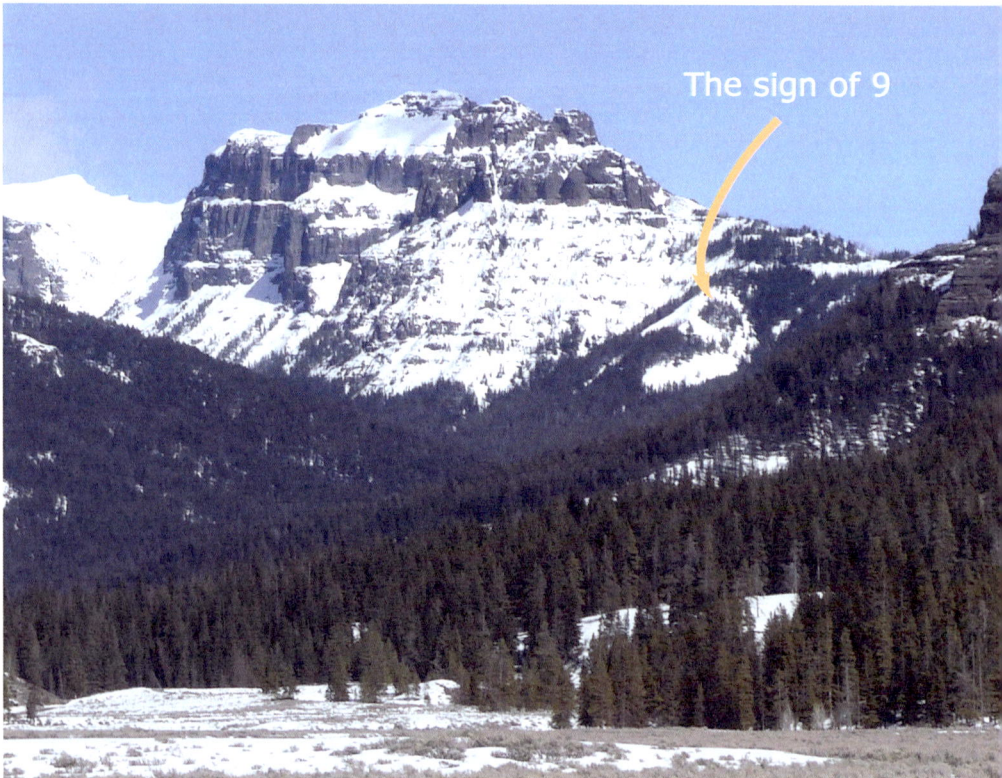

The sign of 9

Wolf #9

Wolf #9 was the **o**rig**i**nal "Eve" of the **Yel**l**ow**st**o**ne wolves. **A**long with her **daugh**ter, Wolf #7, sh**e** was **a**mong the first 14 wolves **re**intr**o**d**u**ced to **Yel**l**ow**st**o**ne **Na**tion**a**l Park in **Jan**u**ar**y 1995. **To**d**ay**, a **sig**nifi**c**ant **per**cent**age** of **Yel**l**ow**st**o**ne wolves **ca**rry her g**e**nes.

Every **win**ter, "The S**i**gn of 9" can b**e** s**ee**n on the sl**o**pes of one of the **migh**ty **A**bsar**o**ka **Moun**tains, which **bor**ders the **east**ern end of **La**mar **Val**l**ey**.

This marks the r**ou**te Wolf #9 took to l**e**ave her R**o**se Cr**ee**k Pack and **ven**ture **in**to the w**i**lds of **Wy**o**ming to b**e**come a **found**ing **mem**ber of two more wolf packs: the Clark's Fork and **Bea**rtooth packs. - **L**e**o Leck**i**e

Sound Key

How Noah Text® Works

Noah Text® allows readers to see sound-parts within words, providing a way for struggling readers to decode and enunciate words that are difficult to access. In turn, their improvement in reading accuracy and fluency frees up cognitive resources that they can devote to comprehending the meaning of the text, enabling them to truly enjoy reading while building their reading skills.

Syllables

A *syllable* is a unit of pronunciation with only one vowel sound, with or without surrounding consonants. Syllables line up with the way we speak and are an integrated unit of speech and hearing. Teachers often clap out syllables with their students.

Noah Text® acts upon words with more than one syllable. In a multiple-syllable word, the presentation of each syllable alternates bold, not bold, bold, etc. For example, the word "syllable" would be presented as "**syl**la**ble**," while the word "sound" is not changed at all.

Vowels

A long vowel is a vowel that pronounces its own letter name. Here are some examples of underlined long vowels you will find in Noah Text®, along with syllable breaks that are made obvious:

Long (a)

pl<u>a</u>te, p<u>a</u>in, **hes**i**t<u>a</u>te**, **n<u>a</u>**tion

h<u>a</u>ir, r<u>a</u>re, **par**ent, **l<u>i</u>**br<u>a</u>ry

p<u>a</u>le, f<u>a</u>il, **de**t<u>a</u>il

tr<u>a</u>y, **al**w<u>a</u>ys

Long (e)

feet, teach, **com**plete

feel, deal, **ap**peal

ear, fear, here, **dis**appear, **se**vere

Long (i)

tribe, like, night, **high**light

fire, **ad**mire, **re**quire

mile, pile, **a**while, **rep**tile

Long (o)

globe, nose, suppose, **re**mote

coach, whole, coal, goal, **ap**proach

mow, blown, **win**dow

Long (u)

huge, mule, **fu**el, **per**fume, **a**muse

hue, **ar**gue, **tis**sue, blue, **pol**lution

116

Disclaimer: As noted in the research provided at noahtext.com, the English writing system is extremely complex. Thus, the process of segmenting syllables, identifying rime patterns, and highlighting long vowels, is not only tedious but ambiguous at times based on the pronunciation of various regional dialects, the complexity of English orthography, and other articulatory considerations. Noah Text® strives to be as accurate as possible in developing clear, concise modified text that will assist readers; however, it cannot guarantee universal agreement on how all words are pronounced.

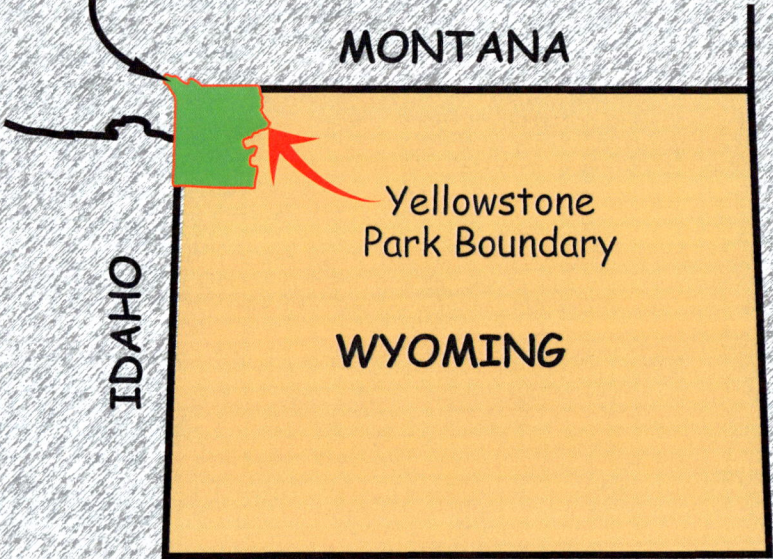

Vocabulary

Anthro**po**mor**phism** - **Giv**ing **hu**man **cha**rac**teristics** to **animals**. Or to **hu**man**ize**.

Aurora **bor**eal**is** - **stre**amers or **arch**es of light that **oc**cur in earth's **north**ern **hem**isph**ere** - called **north**ern lights.

Eradi**cate** - to get rid of **some**thing **com**pl**ete**ly.

Exter**mi**n**ation** - **kill**ing, **es**pe**cial**ly of a wh**ole** gro**up** of **animals**.

Poach**ing** - **ill**e**gal hunt**ing and **cap**tur**ing** of **animals**.

Soci**etal** - **Ac**tions that **re**l**ate** to or **in**volve a **so**ci**ety** (a large gro**up** that **li**ves **to**geth**er**, **de**ci**des** how to do things, and shares the work that n**ee**ds to be done).

Ung**u**late - a hoofed **mam**mal l**i**ke a horse, pig, d**eer**, elk or **bi**son as some **ex**am**ples**.

www.ingramcontent.com/pod-product-compliance
Lightning Source LLC
Chambersburg PA
CBRC090850210326
41597CB00007B/158